# THE BACK BOOK

Also by Cal del Pozo

*Bunnetics: How to Shape Your Buns*
*Twenty Days to a Trimmer Torso*

# THE BACK BOOK

*A Complete Health and Exercise Program
to Cure Your Aching Back*

**Cal del Pozo**

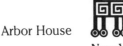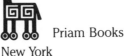

Arbor House     Priam Books
New York

Library of Congress Catalog Card Number: 83-73062

ISBN: 0-87795-515-8
MANUFACTURED IN THE UNITED STATES OF AMERICA
10 9 8 7 6 5 4 3 2 1

This book is printed on acid free paper. The paper in this book meets the guidelines for permanence and durability of the Committee on Production Guidelines for Book Longevity of the Council on Library Resources.

Photos by Ralph Bogertman.

Text design by Antler & Baldwin, Inc.

To be able to spend the major portion of my life doing what I enjoy most, dancing, teaching, and helping other people look and feel better, is a privilege—and one which, for the most part, I owe to those who have been my teachers during these last twenty-five years. Therefore I dedicate this book to one in particular, Ms. Dagmar Jarvel, whose instruction and care I proudly cherish.

# ACKNOWLEDGMENTS

A lot of fruitless time would have been spent in the initial research, the clarification of medical terminology and the final concept and direction of the book had it not been for the time and help of Dr. Carlos Yanez, M.D. in Corpus Christie, Texas and in New York City; Dr. William Hamilton, M.D., Dr. William Nagler, M.D., Dr. Paul Scoles, M.D., Dr. Richard Bachrach, D.O., Dr. Richard Carnival, D.C. and Dr. Jacclyn Robbins, D.C. Also a very special thanks to Tim Pearson, Marilyn DeVoe, Ellaine and Rick Russell, my agent, Ivy Fisher Stone and to my editor at Arbor House, Debbie Wilburn.

# FOREWORD

One of the most frequent complaints physicians hear from their patients has to do with some form of back pain, the cause for which can sometimes challenge the diagnostic and therapeutic skills of even the most experienced of us who treat back patients. Indeed, back problems, regardless of their origin, not only cause a good deal of discomfort, they almost always result in our taking time out from our normal activities. Cal's book initially reminded me of how little in the way of prevention is taught to doctors in training as well as the general public. If more of us would learn how to care for our backs, perhaps fewer of us would experience back problems and subsequently need to rush to a doctor when pain develops. This book helps to fill that void by offering exercises on back-pain prevention as well as sound advice for keeping a strong back healthy. Furthermore, the need for regular strengthening exercises is essential for the patient with chronic back problems, and this cannot be overemphasized. Cal's intrinsic understanding of back problems and the need for structured exercise as provided in the four-week rehabilitative exercise program can be invaluable for such patients.

Cal's first-hand experience in the dance world and his devotion to physical fitness have given him an admirable background and understanding of the back and its related problems. And as he is careful to point out, a prompt and complete medical evaluation is always the first step to recovery for anyone with a painful back. Beyond this, there is no question that strengthening back muscles through exercise will provide a protective support that can ward off many future problems. The approach used in this book to achieve this goal is not only easy to understand, but is delivered with accuracy and concern for the problems of back-pain sufferers.

Remember that it takes effort and patience to have and maintain a healthy back, and it is the responsibility of each of us to maintain its fitness. *The Back Book* should certainly be read by anyone looking for a safe, no-nonsense guide to back care, which will result in a healthier back and, consequently, a healthier life. I encourage you to use it and enjoy the benefits it can bring.

—Carmen A. Cross, M.D.

# CONTENTS

# SECTION THREE

# INTRODUCTION

Professional dancers are considered to be among the most physically fit athletes in the world. Dance is, after all, exercise in its purest and most rhythmically controlled form. The noted choreographer and dance historian Agnes de Mille wrote in *The Book of the Dance*, "A dancer is special—his body is not like ours—he can do things we can't."

Dancers always place unnatural demands on their bodies, especially in performance. The ever present competitive attitude, the strive for performance excellence and the energy received from knowing that one is being watched results in a dancer putting his or her body through tremendous levels of exertion in seconds. But the physical risks a dancer takes are similar to those experienced by others who participate in activities requiring a great deal of energy and physical exertion. The most common injuries suffered include torn ligaments, pulled muscles, inflammation of tendons and joint sprains. When it comes to back trouble, dancers usually have complications involving fractures of the vertebral transverse and spinous processes—a hazard of the trade which they share with other athletes whose sport involves back bends and high leg extensions.

Generally speaking, though, dancers usually don't suffer from back pain since they spend the major part of their lives toning their muscles and indirectly caring for their backs by developing abdominal strength and muscular properties, such as elasticity and contractability. These are an integral part of dance training and technique, but are also the basic ingredients for a healthy back.

I have been a dancer for twenty-five years, and as all dancers I have always been proud of my ability to make my body move in ways it isn't even designed to move. So why, you might ask at this point, is a dancer writing a book about back care?

Because even though I am in good shape, I am also a prime example of the fact that backs don't just turn against the overweight, the sedentary, the aging, or the underexercised. Everybody is a candidate for back pain; in fact it is estimated that four out of every five adults will come to know how painfully stubborn their backs can be at least once in their lifetime. I belong to that group.

One evening while on stage I suffered a bad fall which sent agonizing pain up and down my back. I had to be carried to the hospital. There I was told that although I had landed on my tail bone, my spine was fine. Instead, I had dislocated my right leg from the hip socket and torn both hamstring muscles with such force that it had provoked a stress fracture of the right hip bone. Muscle relaxers and complete bed rest were the prescription and for six months I did nothing but catch up on the television industry.

In my eagerness to return to dance I didn't listen to my doctor's advice to return to my old routine gradually. I went back into training as if nothing had happened. Why not? I reasoned that I was young, I felt good. I was in good shape. Soon I found that being in good shape does not last forever, or even for a short time. After less than three weeks of training my body rebelled in the form of renewed back pain. My muscles had lost their tone. It took me a year to gradually get back into shape and to relieve the pain— and the fear of it—that goes with it.

During that year I devised a series of exercises, some based on standard exercises prescribed for back care and rehabilitation and some based on techniques of dance and Yoga. I talked to every physician who specialized in back care who could give me some of his or her time. Many did. It is through their cooperation that I have been able to compile much of the information found in this book.

Today I devote a great deal of time to teaching adults how to get into and stay in shape. Back care is always emphasized in my exercises. And even though I am a little older and my body can no longer perform the feats it once did, through these exercises I have been able to keep my back and those of the students I teach strong and trouble-free.

I realize that in your quest for relief of back pain chances are this is not the first back book you have read. The exercises in this book can do much to strengthen your back and relieve pain. But a lot depends on you. The exercises must be done regularly and correctly, and you'll find as you read on that the directions have been carefully written to insure that they will be properly executed. If you take the time and make the effort, you'll soon find how easy it is to take care of your back and free yourself from a life of worry, unnecessary medical expense and needless limitation of your physical activities. This is the intended goal of the book and my final reason for writing it.

—Cal del Pozo

# SECTION

1

# DOCTORS
# AND EXERCISE

Statistics show that doctors receive more complaints about back pain than any other single ailment, with the exception of respiratory infection. And just as there are hundreds of myths and home cures for the common cold, there are as many for back-related problems. And they keep coming, from boots that allow you to hang upside down to fancy battery-operated machines that resemble a Ferris wheel. While many of these inventions may offer temporary relief for some, research studies show that a painful back does not go away without proper medical attention, care and proper exercise.

Fortunately, most physicians are quick to agree that proper body mechanics and exercise are the best preventive medicine and cure for most causes of back pain. But exercise also has its drawbacks. Although doctors frequently recommend exercise to their patients, few have the time or the knowledge to teach people how to exercise and how much exercise is enough or too much. In our present concern for trimmed bodies, cardio-vascular endurance and longevity, there are those who will exercise to the point of total fatigue. Too much exercise, especially when you have a back condition, is as bad or worse than no exercise at all. Exercise must be planned and studied before execution. The more information you have about your body's requirements, capabilities and limits, the better you will be able to choose the correct exercise system. When it comes to a bad back, exercise must be approached in stages. The first stage must be one of rehabilitation as you learn about your back and what has caused the malfunction while giving your back muscles time to release their painful tension. The second stage involves gradual regaining of strength and flexibility, and the third stage involves more rigorous exercise to develop additional strength, elasticity and endurance. *The Back Book: A Complete Health and Exercise Program to Cure Your Aching Back* is divided into three sections, covering each of these stages.

When done with your doctor's consent, the exercises in this book can guide you toward a healthier body and a stronger back. And although its primary objective is to help you get back on your feet pain-free, it is not purported to be a miracle cure book, nor can it possibly apply to every kind of back trouble. But if you give yourself the time to read and follow its instructions, chances are you will reap tremendous benefits.

# BACK PAIN

Back pain—it is painful. Redundant, yes; obvious, yes. To make matters worse, back pain is often hard to localize or measure and frequently it goes away as suddenly as it hits. Whether it hits you for the first time or the fourth, two things are certain: one, the causes of back pain are complex and two, back pain, when recurrent or acute, should never be left medically unattended. In most cases when back pain strikes there is usually no reason for alarm. After a few days of bed rest the pain will disappear. This is both a good and a bad characteristic: it is good because the aches and frustrations cease, but it is bad because too many people cancel or fail to show up for the doctor's appointment they made when the pain first hit. At the risk of sounding like a nagging parent, not seeing a doctor even if the pain subsides after a few days could be a grave mistake and one for which you might pay serious consequences.

## WHEN BACK PAIN HITS

When back pain hits, especially if it hits acutely, even the calmest people become irritated and nervous. This is not to say that that is an unnatural reaction, but let me remind you that nervous stress, in itself a cause of back pain, will only add to your present discomfort. When pain hits try to relax and do two things:
1) Call your doctor. If you don't have one look in your telephone directory for the local chapter of the American Medical Association. They will provide you with the names of a couple of specialists in your area.
2) Don't try to be your own diagnostician. Often the simplest forms of back pain, such as muscle spasm, present symptoms similar to other problems that are more complicated. In just a few minutes on the phone your doctor can sort them out. But don't take risks by not contacting him or her.

## CONSULTING WITH YOUR DOCTOR

If you have been involved in an accident or if your pain followed any kind of unusual physical exertion, tell the doctor immediately. Otherwise let him ask the questions. He will probably first want to know your age and if you have a history of back trouble.

Dr. William Hamilton, an orthopedic consultant with the New York City Ballet and a man who has helped thousands of athletes and dancers, myself included, advises to be prepared to answer the following questions which doctors frequently ask:

1. How long have you been in pain?
2. Do you have a fever?
3. Does the pain go down your legs?
4. Do you feel weakness or numbness in the leg muscles or feet?
5. Are you experiencing any difficulty urinating or having a bowel movement?

According to Dr. Hamilton, a yes answer to any of those questions is an alert that a "red flag" condition may be present and the patient will be asked to come in for an examination. If leg pain is not present but the person is older and the pain is persistent, the patient will also be asked to come into the office.

Once there, the first thing the doctor will do is get a complete medical history. Dr. Richard Bachrach, a New York City osteopath to whom many orthopedics refer their back patients, explained that the root of the problem normally comes out in that conversation—an accident you might have had years ago which may not have required treatment then may be an important link to discovering the cause of your current difficulty.

## BED REST

We all know that getting an immediate appointment with a doctor is not always possible. He or she will most likely ask you to stay in bed for a few days. Bed rest is always great on a Sunday morning with the newspaper and a cup of freshly brewed coffee in hand, but not so great when it is mandatory and you feel you can't even reach for a coffee mug, let alone open a newspaper. The following guidelines will help you not only to get the best from your time in bed, but to relax and alleviate some of that pain.

1. Bed rest means stay in bed. Spend a few moments thinking of all the things you might need and make them accessible to your reach. Avoid having to get in and out of bed.

2. A firm mattress is what you should be lying on. If you don't have one and can't get someone to provide you with a board that can be placed

under your mattress, your best bet is to get some help and place the mattress on the floor. You could also throw a few blankets onto the floor and use that as your bed. The problem with this alternative is that getting up from the floor to go to the bathroom, for instance, can aggravate your pain further. Crawling on all fours would be your least painful choice for getting around. Try the Yellow Pages for listings of companies under Bed-Rentals and Mattresses and Bedding. Prices will vary according to your area, but it would be worth checking into renting a posturepedic bed or mattress. Some insurance companies will cover a portion of this expense if it is medically prescribed.

3. While in bed there are two body positions that are the most recommended:

The V or Semisitting Position: As illustrated, place a pillow under the knees to keep them elevated at a 90 degree angle, and place a pillow or a bunch of them behind your back and neck to keep your upper torso at a ninety degree angle with your thighs. This position will keep your hip flexor muscles in a relaxed state and reduce their pull on the pelvic area. It will also help to increase the space between the lumbar vertebrae, relieving pressure on nerves that might be pinched.

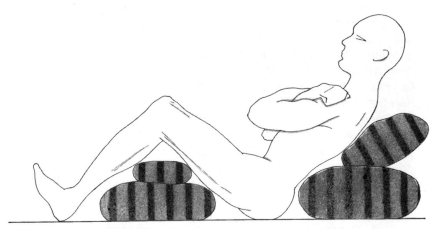

The Fetal Position: Lying on one side, bring your knees and chest toward one another. The upper knee should rest on the mattress slightly higher than the other. A pillow between both legs will help to make this position easier. Put a small pillow on the resting side of your head to keep it in alignment with your spine.

Rolling from one side to another without help can be a painful ordeal. It can be done with a minimum of discomfort if you do it in the following manner:

1. Place your upper hand on the mattress, close to the body at mid-chest level.

2. Take a deep breath. Hold it for a second or two and picture yourself pushing with your hand against the mattress, then rolling first your knees, followed immediately by your hips and torso until you are on your back, with knees bent, facing the ceiling. As you exhale, push and do just that.

3. While facing the ceiling, cross your arms across your chest and take a deep breath. Hold it for a second or two and exhale as slowly as you can while concentrating on letting the knees, then the hips, torso and head roll to the other side.

Be aware that what makes this change of position easier to accomplish is the correlation between breathing and picturing in your mind the movement you are going to do before actually executing it. The theory behind this is called ideokinesis or imagined action, which is frequently used in the teaching of correct posture. Imagined Action is discussed in more detail later in this section.

## TENSION-RELEASE EXERCISES DURING BED REST

During the first couple of days the less movement your body is subjected to the better it will be for you. According to Dr. William Nagler, a physiatrist and head of the physical therapy department at New York Hospital, total lack of mobility also has its risks: Tension in the muscles, after a couple of days of immobility, is likely to develop, and as you begin to feel better you might get up too soon. This could cause your rested but weakened muscles to react to their sudden call to action in the form of renewed pain. Sometimes this second attack will hurt even more than the first and you could find yourself right back in bed for an even longer period of time.

If you live alone be sure to take your time in getting up—even if you feel marvelous! Take your first few steps carefully and don't hesitate to hold onto walls and furniture for support. You might feel a slight dizziness and lack of balance after you first get up, or you might feel it when you least expect it. This is a normal reaction coming from your nervous and circulatory systems. Your muscle engine needs a gradual boost after being idle for a while. For better and safer functioning take it slow and easy. Again, do not take unnecessary risks!

The following exercises done over a three-day period are designed to release tensed muscles, activate circulation with a minimum amount of movement and avoid further tension of major muscles that have been inactive. Although I have divided them over a three-day period you can spread them over a longer period if you want. If your pain is acute you will find that the exercises for Day One will be all you can do for a few days. Your body will tell you when to progress to Day Two and Three of the exercises.

**Day One**

Although you won't feel like doing much of anything, this breathing exercise is easy to do and will be very beneficial.

1. While sitting in the V Position pick a spot in the room and focus on it.

2. Slowly wrap your arms across the chest and take a deep breath through your nose. You should feel your stomach swell first, then your rib cage will expand, pushing your arms upward. Hold your breath and count to five.

3. Keeping your eyes focused on the fixed point you have selected, start to count backward from five as you exhale through the mouth. In your mind you must think that the air from your lungs will reach that fixed point by count one.

4. Repeat the same process four more times, trying to take longer each time to exhale. The slower you do it the more relaxed you will become. As tension leaves your arms they will tend to slide down to your sides. Let them.

WARM BATHS AND HEATING PADS

Heat induces the muscles and their nerve end attachments to relax and increases circulation to the areas to which it is applied. But heat should not be applied if your pain is accompanied by an inflammation or discoloration of tissues. This is an indication that your condition could be more than a simple case of muscle spasm.

In cases where none of the Red Flag Alert symptoms mentioned earlier appear, the use of a moist heating pad applied to the most painful area can be of great help. If you feel you hurt all over (physicians call it referred pain), apply it to the lower back area. Most of the main nerves travel to this area and the heat, applied while in the V Sitting Position, will subsequently help to relax them.

Although the benefits of dry heat versus moist heat are controversial, most physicians recommend moist heat. If you have sensitive skin dry heat can produce burns and lesions.

HOT AND COLD PACKS

If your back pain is the result of an injury suffered during sports practice, from a car accident or a fall and you find areas on your back that have swollen, discolored or both, ask your doctor before applying heat. He may recommend that you wait 42 hours before starting alternating applications of heat and cold.

TUB BATHS

If pain is really acute you should not leave bed for the first couple of days other than to go to the bathroom. Taking a couple of warm, not hot water tub baths can make you feel better. It is best to take one in the morning and the other in the late afternoon.

While in the tub do the Tension Release Exercise for Day One. It will be helpful if your tub has one of those non-slip bath mats. It is not only recommended for safety, but will make your V Sitting Position steadier and stop your body from slipping under the water.

**Day Two: Total Body Relaxation**

If, by the end of the first day you still feel pain at the slightest movement, continue to do the Day One exercise. Your body will tell you when it's ready for Day Two.

The object of these exercises is to get you to relax your entire body, a step at a time. They should be done every other hour, alternating with the simple exercise you did on Day One.

*Preparation*: As you see in the illustration the body has been divided into five sections. Section 1 is composed of the feet and ankles; Section 2 the legs and calves; Section 3, the thighs and pelvis; Section 4, the torso and arms (which are wrapped around the chest); Section 5, the shoulders and head.

Each section is further divided into twenty counts. The object is to coordinate your breathing (both inhaling and exhaling) with the counts allocated for each segment of the body. This is done while you continue to

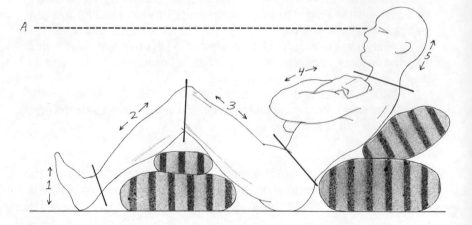

concentrate on the fixed point you selected in the first exercise. After you've gone through the exercise starting with the feet and ankles you will repeat the process in reverse, starting with your head. This exercise can easily be done alone or with someone else counting while you concentrate on the sections that correspond to each series of counts.

The first five counts are always for the slow intake of air through the nose. The following five counts are for the expulsion of air through the mouth. Therefore you will be inhaling during every other set of five counts and exhaling on every other set of five. In addition you must concentrate on the specific section you are working on (feet, legs, thighs, etc.) while inhaling, then concentrate on relaxing that section while exhaling.

*Example*:

Section One (Feet and Ankles), Counts 1 through 20.

1 to 5: To help concentration, look at the fixed point. Breathe in while concentrating on the ankles.

6 to 10: Keep looking at the fixed point. Exhale slowly while trying to relax the feet and ankles. Remember to imagine that the air is reaching the fixed point.

11 to 15: Same as 1 to 5.

16 to 20: Same as 6 to 10.

Repeat the above steps with each section of the body.

Reverse Action (from head to feet).

1 to 5: Exhale as you try to relax the head and all the facial muscles. Close your eyes and do the exercise in reverse, counting backwards.

6 to 10: Inhale and concentrate on the passage of air through the nose.

11 to 15: Exhale and concentrate on further relaxing the head, neck and shoulders. Try to imagine the release of tension traveling down toward the chest.

Now that you have an idea of how it works, try it. You should feel the difference in your body as tension is released. Proper breathing, con-structive relaxation exercises and positive thinking should help get you up and around in no time. But remember, getting out of bed is only the first step toward rehabilitation. Starting an exercise schedule as outlined in Section Two is the second step, while good body mechanics and postural habits comprise the final step to total recovery. All these elements go together hand in hand.

### Day Three: Isometrics

Isometric exercises have been used by physiologists and physical therapists for years in developing muscle strength. Today, even exercise machines are based on isometric principles. "Iso" means equal, while "metrics" means same. In isometric exercises the object is to apply pressure against an immobile object by a major muscle group. It can also be done by applying pressure between two opposing muscle groups, such as the arms, or by tightening or contracting a group of muscles and holding the contraction for a few seconds.

The object of the isometric exercises for Day Three is not to develop strength, but to try to prevent your present muscular strength from decreasing too rapidly during bed rest. To achieve this the exercises will use a minimum amount of pressure. These exercises follow the same counting format as in Day Two. The degree to which you contract your muscles will be light and will be limited to the time it takes to exhale.

These exercises should only be done twice throughout the day. The best times are in the morning and in the evening, before you take your warm tub bath. If you experience any kind of pain when doing these, stop and do not continue. Stick to Day Two. *If your back pain radiates to the buttocks or the legs you should not do Day Three exercises.*

In doing these exercises, as well as when doing others found throughout this book, deep breathing is essential.

We will continue to divide the body into five segments and to allocate twenty counts to each segment. You need not concentrate on the "fixed point" for these exercises. Instead I am going to ask you to concentrate on articulation joints, or, more specifically, segments that connect your body, primarily those in the lower half; think of the ankle joint which connects the feet to the leg; the knee joint which connects the leg to the thigh and the hip joint which connects the thigh to the pelvis.

Although the exercises will concentrate on the arms and the lower limbs, you will also work the chest and shoulders. The neck area, from which a major ramification of the spinal nerves travels to the arms and back, will get the least work. This is a sensitive area, especially if you have developed a stiff neck as a result of muscle spasm in the back or due to bed rest. The exercises for Days One and Two should have helped relieve some of the tension in that area.

Again, keep the pressure light and constant. Concentrate only on the area being worked on. If you feel any indication of discomfort while contracting, stop, relax for a few seconds and go on to the next section.

*Preparation*: Sit in the V Position with your feet and knees close together. Place the palm of your hands on each thigh. Section One (Feet and Ankles), Counts 1 through 20.

1 to 5: Inhale through your nose for the five counts while concentrating on your ankle joints.

6 to 10: On the sixth count flex your ankles by bringing the toes toward you. Exhale slowly through the mouth. Hold your feet in the flexed position

throughout the next four counts. (This will help to stretch the calf muscles and the Achilles tendons which can get stiff during bed rest.)

11 to 15: On the eleventh count point your toes. Inhale slowly. Hold your feet in a pointed position through the next four counts, but do not point your toes too hard. Doing so could cramp the calf muscles.

16 to 20: On the sixteenth count relax the feet. Exhale slowly.

Section Two (Legs)

1 to 5: Inhale slowly and bring your legs and knees close together.

6 to 10: On the sixth count press both of your legs together and sustain the pressure for the next four counts as you exhale.

11 to 15: On the eleventh count release the pressure and inhale slowly.

16 to 20: Repeat the pressure as you exhale.

Section Three (Thighs)

1 to 5: Inhale slowly, make sure your hands are placed on top of each thigh.

6 to 10: On the sixth count lightly press your right hand against your right thigh. At the same time slide your right foot back a couple of inches toward your pelvis. Press thigh and hand together with light force. Maintain this isometric contraction throughout your four counts of exhalation.

11 to 15: Release the contraction as you inhale. Slide the foot back down, resting the thigh on the pillow underneath.

Repeat the exercise on the left side.

Section Four (Buttocks and Stomach)

1 to 5: Use these counts to take a deep breath.

6 to 10: On the sixth count tighten your buttock muscles as firmly as you can and hold the contraction throughout the five counts as you exhale.

11 to 15: Release the contraction and inhale deeply.

16 to 20: On the sixteenth count tighten your lower stomach as firmly as possible and hold for five counts as you exhale.

Section Five (Chest, Shoulders and Neck)

1 to 5: Lift both arms over your head as high as you can as you inhale while dropping your head down to your chest.

6 to 10: As you exhale let your head drop back so that you're looking at the ceiling and bring your arms down so that your elbows touch. The lower arms will open sideways, forming a wide V. The upper back will develop a slight roundness.

11 to 15: Repeat counts 1 to 5.

16 to 20: Repeat counts 6 to 10.

Do the set of exercises once again, in reverse order.

# UNDERSTANDING BACK PAIN

Among the various combinations of bones, muscles and connective tissues that form the supportive structure of the human body, the spine reigns as its architectural wonder. While the heart is the muscle that pumps life to our bodies and the brain is our center of command, the spine is the center of operation from which all movements involving the upper and lower limbs are directed. In fact the spine is so functionally prolific that there are few movements that can be executed without some degree of spinal involvement. Because the back is so intimately connected to the rest of the body, learning about how it functions is beneficial to it as a whole. This chapter contains general information about the spine which I believe to be necessary for the protection and maintenance of a pain-free back.

When the engine in a car malfunctions, lifting the hood to see what is wrong is of little use unless you understand the purpose of the different tubes and wires and of the parts they connect. And even if you are somewhat familiar with the engine, chances are you would still need a mechanic to help you correct the problem. But not even an expert mechanic can guarantee permanent results if the car's malfunction was related to the fuel you used and you continue to use it, or because of poor driving habits which weren't corrected. You will inevitably end up with the car in the garage again.

The same applies to your back—your knowledge of its working parts and their limitations, your ability to communicate with your physician and the manner in which you follow, or don't follow his advice, are what can start you on a trouble-free road much faster and without fear of future complications. The health of your back largely depends on you and the efforts you're willing to make in caring for it.

## THE SPINE

The spine is a skeletal column formed by thirty-three (or thirty-four) small bones called vertebrae, which are separated and cushioned by fluid-

26

filled oval pads called discs. The spine's primary function is that of supporting the body's weight. Movement is its secondary function. When looked at from behind, the normal spine presents its vertebrae in a straight line from the base of the skull to its tapered end, called the coccyx or tail bone. But from a side view it shows that the vertebrae form a series of curves—five in total—which are responsible for the spine's weight support function. This responsibility is made possible by the way the curves are arranged (two forward and three backward) and by the number and structure of the vertebrae found in each curve.

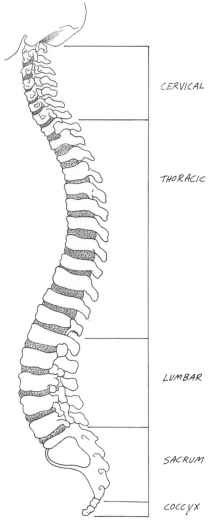

CERVICAL

THORACIC

LUMBAR

SACRUM

COCCYX

*A lateral view of the spine and its five curves. Cervical (seven vertebrae); Thoracic (twelve vertebrae); Lumbar (five vertebrae); Sacrum (five vertebrae); Cocyx (four or five vertebrae). Note how the two forward curves, the cervical and the lumbar, have the smallest and largest vertebrae, respectively. These areas also have the most mobility; as a result back pain frequently manifests itself here.*

From the head down they are: The cervical curve (neck region: seven vertebrae); the thoracic or dorsal curve (chest region: twelve vertebrae); and the lumbar curve (low back region: five vertebrae). The fourth and fifth curve represent the immobile regions of the spine. They are formed by the sacrum (five vertebrae that are fused together into one unit) and the coccyx (four or at times five vertebrae).

The spine also assists in the maintenance of the erect posture, although the correctness of posture is determined by the combined efforts of the muscles, the alignment of the vertebrae and the execution of body mechanics. In addition, the spine encases and protects the spinal cord and acts as the body's axle. Its vertebrae function as the body's strongest shock absorbers.

### Mobility

The spine has more mobility as a unit than it has in its individual sections. In these sections movement between the vertebrae is determined by bony spurs called facet joints which articulate with each other. These joints are what you hear snap when you twist your torso or when a chiropractor or osteopath applies manipulative pressure. Strangely enough, freedom of overall spinal movement is greater in those curves where the vertebrae are smaller, such as in the neck or cervical region, or larger, such as in the lumbar region. Because of the mobility of these two areas, they are the most prone to injury. The spinal curves allow the spine to bend forward (flex) and backward (extend). It can also bend from side to side (lateral flexion), rotate (twist), and roll clockwise and counterclockwise (circumvent). The above-mentioned movements performed by the spine involve large areas of muscle. They also happen to be movements that either are not common in most people's daily routine, or when they are common are not performed to their fullest extent. Muscles get out of shape, or even atrophied, when the actions they are designed to perform are not executed often, or at all. Therefore unless such movements are integrated into a person's physical routine, especially as years progress, the musculature of the back will weaken. When they are called to perform any of those actions, as simple as they may seem, their backs become susceptible to injuries. Ligament tears and muscle pulls or spasms are the most common and painful. As you will see in Sections Two and Three, many of the exercises for maintenance of a healthy back are based on the same movements that are characteristic of the spine's mechanical function.

### Miscellaneous Causes of Spinal-Related Pain

It is a rare occurrence when back pain is brought on by spinal causes only. Normally other factors are involved, either from the nervous system (i.e., stress) or the muscular system (i.e., pulled muscle or spasm) or a traumatic incident, such as an accident. The spine is well protected, and because the muscular system is so intimately involved with it, back pain— of which lower back pain is the most common—is either of a muscular nature or a combination of muscular and skeletal causes.

In relation to the spine, back pain can result if something interferes with the spine's ability to support the body's weight properly. What could cause such interference? It could be caused by lack of flexibility in the chest and rib cage, which is frequently found in people who overwork the muscles in that area, such as weight lifters. Another cause could be muscle tension and lack of flexibility in the upper chest, shoulders and neck, due to the postural habit of allowing the head to jut forward, which would put it out of alignment with the spine.

But probably the worst offender in obstructing the spine's weight supporting function is the psoas major muscles, commonly referred to as the illiopsoas. This long pair of muscles originates at both sides of the last thoracic vertebra and the first four lumbar vertebrae, and attach to the thighs. Their prolonged state of contraction, which occurs among people who must sit for long periods of time, results in tightness at the hip joints, thigh and hamstring muscles. This tends to alter a person's postural habits and, thus, the alignment of his or her spine. In addition, the illipsoas take direct part in the forward bending of the torso, movements of the legs, rotation of the pelvis and many other movements that are common to our daily mechanical habits. Because of the variety of roles these muscles play in our daily lives, their conditioning is essential to proper alignment of the spine, which they can influence more than any other structure in our bodies. Oddly enough most exercise systems, including the most popular ones, do not stress proper conditioning of these muscles. According to Dr. Bachrach, whose practice includes many famous dancers and athletes, the vast majority of the cases he treats, not just for low back pain but pain affecting the hips, knees, upper back, neck, feet and ankles, are caused by tightness of this muscle.

Other problems we have with our spines—if they're not related to a muscular condition—are caused by its components, specifically the vertebrae and their discs. Since these, in turn, are often attached to ligaments, muscles, or both, which are then connected to nerves, anything that can go wrong with any one of these components will ultimately involve all of them. Therefore, starting with the vertebrae, let's take a brief look at their structure and their most common relation to back pain.

### Vertebrae
A vertebra is structurally divided into two main sections: the body or

front, which is the bulkiest section, and the back section or vertebral arch. The body resembles a flat drum and acts as the main bearer of weight. The vertebral body is connected to the vertebral arch by two bony extensions (one on each side), called the pedicles. These three structures, the body, the pedicles jutting from both sides of the body and the vertebral arch, form the walls of the canal that houses the spinal cord. The odd projections seen in vertebrae are called processes. There are seven of them, some of which are attached to muscles and ligaments. They provide the spine with support and overall flexibility.

Of the seven processes, three of them (the largest ones) give a vertebra the look of a three-pronged crown. Of these, the two lateral or transverse processes, which travel outward and sideways from the arch, are the most

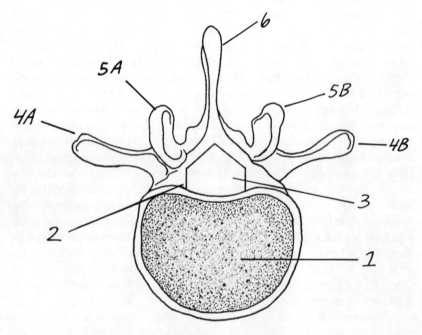

*A superior view of a lumbar vertebrae.*
1. *The vertebral body*
2. *The Pedicle which connects the vertebral body*
   *to the vertebral arch*
*2 through 6: The vertebral arch*
3. *The spinal canal*
*4A and 4B. The transverse process*
*5A and 5B. The facet joints*
6. *The spinous process*

prone to fractures. The transverse processes of one vertebra connect with those of the vertebrae above and below at the points where they emerge from the vertebral arch. These junctures form small openings called the spinal foramina, through which exit pairs of main nerves coming from the spinal cord. In case of fracture or other causes (such as the ones listed under Mechanical Disorders) the foramen could narrow, pressing the nerves they protect, resulting in pain. If the nerve being "pinched" is the main one, or if it, and its ramifications, travel great distances in the body, pain can be felt throughout an entire area, making it difficult to locate the origin of the pain. Located between the transverse process is the spinous process, which points downward toward the pelvis. It is the spinous process that forms that chain of bumps that can be seen and felt when you run your hand up and down the back. The length of the spinous process in an individual largely determines the degree to which one's back can bend backward. Dancers and gymnasts who perform backbends routinely are prone to fractures of these protuberances. So are swimmers who special-ize in the back or butterfly stroke. Football players are also prone to spinous process injury. Children have been known to sustain process fractures which can go undetected for years. Whenever young children complain of back pain, they should be seen by a doctor immediately, especially if they are active children or involved in any of these sports. Although the spinous processes may seem very close to the skin, they are actually located between half an inch and two inches below the skin's surface, depending on the person's size and weight. That is why on a thin person an on-sight examination of the spine can provide a relatively accurate impression of the person's spinal alignment, while on people who are overweight or obese X-rays might be necessary before diagnosis, even when the causes of pain may not seem alarming or due to trauma, such as an accident.

### Facet Joints

If you have been to a chiropractor or an osteopathic physician who has manipulated your back, or if you have ever heard a cracking sound when twisting your torso, you have been "talked to" by a facet joint. They are located in pairs above and below each vertebra and interlock with the processes of their adjoining neighbors. Facet joints are like the hinges of the spine and are capped and oiled by a smooth white cartilage tissue that permits their movement. The facet joints are extremely important in the alignment of the spinal column. They are as strong as they are small.

Although facet joints can easily get out of alignment by either skeletal unbalance or muscular unbalance (such as when there is muscle spasm on one side of the spine), it would be easier to dislocate an arm than it would be to dislocate a facet joint. Still, misalignment can result from bad posture, the aging process or extreme pressure caused by incorrect walking and prolonged incorrect sitting, movements characteristic of some sports that feature constant twisting and bending, and overall bad body mechanics. Through the aging process facet joints can wear and tear and become roughened, allowing the vertebrae they protect to grind against each other. This causes intermittent pain. A perfectly healthy facet joint can, when out of alignment, press a nerve or irritate a ligament. This will also cause back pain and can, for the most part, be remedied through expert manipulation. Although having your back "cracked" feels good and has a certain placebo effect even when cracking is not needed, don't let anyone other than an expert try to crack your back. You'd be surprised how many people have ended up in back braces and traction because of a friendly crack.

### Discs

Discs are the most well-known of the spine's components. They are cushiony oval pads of fibrous cartilage tissue that are located between

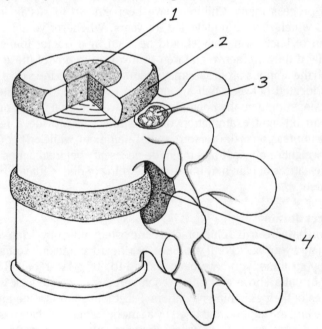

1. The nucleus pulposus
2. The anulus fibrosus
3. The spinal canal
4. The spinal foraminae

each vertebra. While discs separate the vertebrae from one another and contribute to the mobility of the spine, they are also that part of the spine which bears the bulk of the upper body's weight—they are the spine's built-in shock absorbers.

A disc consists of a tough shell, the anulus fibrous formed by layers of overlapping and crisscrossing cartilage fibers. This composition is what allows for the slight mobility between adjacent vertabrae, for that between the spinal curves and, subsequently, for that of the entire spine. The shell contains the disc's fluid, which is mostly water. Each disc has a soft, jellylike center called the nucleus pulposus. It is this center that can often leak through the rear end of the anulus, herniate and cause pressure on the spinal cord.

Discs are in constant action. During the day they are continuously squeezed by the spine's weight-bearing action. That pressure is only reduced during sleep, when the discs reassume their normal size. This is the reason why you are taller in the morning than at the end of the day. The aging process tends to decrease the disc's percentage of fluid and at the same time increase the thickness of the constricting outer shell. This is another reason why we lose a certain amount of elasticity and flexibility as we get older, but the effects needn't be devastating to our health. As Dr. Nagler states, "Older people who eat properly and exercise regularly can beat many of the odds of the aging process and live a long and healthy life with less chances of back trouble and less loss of flexibility."

DISC PROBLEMS

In the lumbar region, where the vertebrae are largest, uneven, persistent pressure felt in a disc can cause a rupture in it. Aside from a direct blow or accident a rupture or herniation can be prompted by habitually bad posture, poor muscle tone, ligament strain or any condition promoting bad spinal alignment. Bulging, ruptures or herniations have more chance of happening in a disc that has already been weakened by pathological conditions. But these problems, I must emphasize, are extremely low on the long list of causes of back pain. Discs are not fragile structures.

Unfortunately, when back pain hits most people immediately think the worst—slipped disc. Discs can experience several traumatic conditions, the most common being that of fluid leaking out, but the disc itself cannot slip out.

What could cause a disc to leak? The pressure inside a disc is calculated at about 100 pounds per square inch. The constant pressurized action of the fluid is what actually helps to keep the vertebrae apart and prevents them from grinding against one another. The fluid is constantly being replenished by the flow of body nutrients, primarily plasma, which reaches a spongelike cartilage that separates the disc's center from the vertebral body. This cartilage has several openings through which the plasma travels to keep it healthy and alive. When, due to accidental injury or pathological cause, this interchange of fluid is impaired, the cartilage can swell or break. The disc in turn can also swell, degenerate, displace or disintegrate. In such cases the vertebrae, less their cushiony buffer, can rub together and press or "pinch" nerve roots, causing extreme pain. When this happens, time and rest are the only remedy.

Swelling in a disc can cause additional problems: when a disc swells, the pressure of its fluid increases and the tension can cause tearing, bleeding and swelling of surrounding structures like ligaments. This can be accompanied by severe muscle spasms which, besides being quite painful, will restrict mobility to the area and possibly in surrounding areas. This can result in added stiffness, more pain and, needless to say, tremendous frustration. In such cases, bed rest is the most frequently prescribed "medication" to alleviate the tension and allow the swelling to subside.

There are rare instances when the swelling of a disc may not respond to bed rest. The disc might even rupture or burst, and fragments of it could lodge themselves in the membranes of the spinal canal. Frequently a nerve root will be compressed because of the continuous swelling, and pain will be felt in the areas covered by that nerve and its ramifications. In this case your doctor might resolve to call in a surgeon to relieve the pressure, which should help get you back on your feet in no time. Gradual exercise should then be started to rehabilitate and strengthen the ligaments and muscles following your recovery period.

SCIATICA

Sometimes a bulging disc, specifically from either the fourth and fifth lumbar vertebrae or the first three sacral vertebrae, will cause pressure on the main nerves connected to these vertebrae. These nerves join together to form the sciatic nerve, which is the longest in the body. Ramifications of the sciatic nerve cover the buttocks and the legs. Pressure on this nerve at its origin, or even abnormal sensations received by its ramifications, can produce pain and tightness in one or both limbs. So sensitive is the sciatic nerve that even sitting on a wallet carried in the back pocket can often be the culprit behind minor sciatic conditions.

Sciatic pain can sometimes be strong enough to keep a person off his or her feet completely. Rest, careful stretching of the lower back, buttocks and leg muscles, and proper posture are the best way to alleviate this condition. It should be noted that most cases of sciatic pain are not related to disc problems, but can be traced to muscle spasm or bad alignment of the facet joints between the sacrum and the fifth lumbar vertebra, or among the lumbar vertebrae themselves. In this case manipulation techniques are used to relieve both muscular and nerve tension. Because the symptoms of sciatica are so similar to those of other back problems, only medical examination can determine if a disc is actually the culprit.

### The Swaying Pelvis

There is no other part of the skeletal structure that has as much importance or influence on both the spine and back pain as the pelvis. Even when problems originate in the upper regions of the spine, in most cases the cause can be traced to the pelvis' alignment in relation to the spine. The pelvis is also important because part of its function is to absorb the shock of weight during movement, and to transfer the weight of the trunk, head and arms to the lower extremities. The back of the pelvis is formed by the sacrum, the fourth section of the spine. The sacrum connects to the upper spine at the lumbosacral joint, which is the spot where the facet joints of the fifth lumbar vertebra connect with the facet joints of the first sacral vertebra. It is at this joint that the spine and pelvis have their greater mobility; consequently it is the spot where the majority of mechanical problems found in our backs originate.

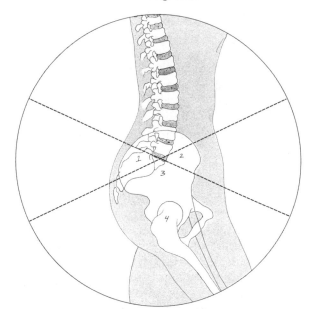

*The Swaying Pelvis*
*1. The sacrum*
*2. The lumbosacral joint, the area where the dotted lines cross.*
*3. The pelvis crest (hip bone)*
*4. The hip joint*

Most mechanical problems are in themselves related to posture. At the lumbosacral joint the pelvis can tilt too far back, increasing the normal forward curvature of the lumbar area causing extreme lordosis or swayback (hyperlordosis). This condition places extreme pressure on the lumbar section, leading to several pain-inducing conditions, such as stress of the vertebrae and their various articulating joints, to bulging of the discs and consequently pressure on the various main nerves of that region, to stretching of the ligaments. Although there may be other problems that contribute to swayback, poor muscle tone and poor posture are the most prevalent causes.

Most of the fifty-seven muscles that are found in the trunk, lower limbs and at the sides of the arms originate at the pelvis. These muscles assist the back in a variety of functions, such as lifting, and are crucial to daily activities such as walking, bending, raising or crossing a leg, etc. In other words, the pelvis is the center of control of body movement and the area where all the balancing forces of the body come together. This is why, as we'll discuss in Section Three, keeping the pelvis centered under the trunk is an integral part of learning correct postural habits and overall movements.

SWAYBACK AND LUMBAR PAIN

Because the lumbar region curves inward, we all naturally have a slight swayback. When that indentation is extreme, problems arise. Extreme swayback or hyperlordosis, which has certain genetic influences, is mainly due to bad postural habits and poor muscle tone. Often swayback is blamed on weak abdominal muscles, but that theory is much like the question of which came first—the chicken or the egg? The main problem arising from extreme swayback is that the various ligaments that reinforce the connection between the pelvis—specifically the sacrum—to the fifth lumbar vertebra must bear too much of the upper body's weight while standing. This can often cause the fifth lumbar vertebra to slip forward. When such a problem arises, Dr. Hamilton states, "A person is practically walking on borrowed time from his facet joints and ligaments," until one day when excruciating lumbar pain hits.

Of the nineteen ligaments that strengthen the junction of the pelvic bones and sacrum with the coccyx, two are the most prone to stress and injury from the slippage of the fifth lumbar vertebra: one is the anterior longitudinal ligament, which runs the entire length of the spine on both sides (anterior and posterior), and is connected to all the vertebrae, their discs and other ligaments; and the ileofemoral ligaments or Y ligaments, which control the forward and backward tilting of the pelvis. This function cannot be performed when the fifth lumbar vertebra is inclined too far forward and the muscles of the lower back and the legs, especially, the hamstring muscles, become very tight.

Other than problems related to the position of the pelvis, which again are mostly postural, pain in the lumbar region can be caused by the combined stress of the illiopsoas, the Y and the longitudinal ligaments due to prolonged sitting, which will cause tightness in the hips and thighs, and by poor sleeping habits.

Sleeping on your back, for example, pulls the Y ligament and thus aggravates the swayback condition. People who sleep in this position could find themselves unable to get out of bed one morning due to pain from muscles that have been strained throughout the night by the pulling force of the Y ligament. Also people who sleep with numerous pillows, a habit which forces the head into a prolonged forward position, can develop tightness in the neck area and can even result in pinched nerves due to forcibly misaligned facet joints in the cervical vertebrae.

One of the most common causes of lumbar pain or strain, also related to the illiopsoas muscles, is found in badly executed exercises, such as sit-ups done with the legs extended, or straight leg raises done on an inclined board. Even those who have developed strong abdominal muscles could find that one day their backs will fight back in the form of pain. There are many ways that people can safely strengthen their abdominal muscles without doing potentially harmful sit-ups and leg raises. Exercises for abdominal strength as well as for correcting swayback are found in Section Two. Another one of my books, *20 Days to a Trimmer Torso* (Simon & Schuster) concentrates on exercises for abdominal strength.

As we've seen, the back's own complexity subjects it to a variety of dangers. Even if you were to memorize every single spinal component there is, it would be no guarantee that such knowledge could deter you from someday developing back pain. If that were the case physicians would be immune to it, and I've seen too many of them in my fitness classes to know that is not the case. What *is* important is that the knowledge you acquire can serve to increase your awareness not only of what can go wrong with your back, but of how to take fewer risks and thus prevent having things go wrong. Furthermore, such awareness can't help but be of tremendous value in the care of your back and in decreasing the fears you might have during a case of back pain.

In the last few pages we have covered the spine's skeletal components, their interrelated functions and their contribution to several causes of pain. But the two most common reasons for back pain are still those related to muscular problems and stress. Because they also happen to be the ones which, through exercise, we can prevent and control, I have saved them for the end of this section.

## THE MUSCLE QUILT

While the spine bears the body's weight in the standing position, it is the layers of its surrounding muscles that allow it to function in that position. There are over 600 skeletal muscles in our bodies, which constitute between 35 and 50 percent of the body's structure. Of that approximate figure the muscles in the area between the neck and the pelvis take the largest share, acting as constant stabilizers against the force of gravity. Muscles function as the body's own engine. If you were to think of your body as a car, the brain would turn on the ignition while muscles would pull, not push, the bones into action. The manner by which they pull us is determined by their various functions and characteristics.

Basically muscles are divided into either voluntary, those we control, or involuntary, those we can't. Then, according to their primary task of moving the joints of the body, they are further classified into agonists, those which carry out the movement; antagonist, those which support the joint in the opposite direction to the movement that is being executed; synergists, which prevent other muscles from moving in a way that would impair a desired action; and stabilizers, which maintain a joint or joints in a given position, regardless of other movements around it. The classification of a muscle changes with the function it is performing at any given time.

### Characteristics of Muscles

A voluntary muscle consists of a series of muscle fibers and muscle spindles which are bound together by connective tissue, called fascia. The bundling of these fibers form the fleshy part of a muscle, called the belly, which ends in a cordlike fibrous band, called the tendon. In most of our body's joints the belly of a muscle is attached to one bone while the tendon passes over the joint to become firmly attached to the adjoining bone. Contraction of the muscle's belly pulls its tendon, which in turn pulls the joint into action.

According to the particular requirements of a muscle and its location, fascia varies in size, fat content and elasticity, but its role is purely mechanical. It holds the muscles in place and acts as their supporting structure. Lack of exercise, or age, can thicken fascia, restricting the muscle's functions and can even alter a person's posture and ability to move. A process called Rolfing, named after its pioneer, Ida Rolf, involves the tearing of thickened fascia to restore muscular efficiency. Although those who administer this treatment, which is painful and expensive, show countless photographs of satisfied customers before and after the Rolfing sessions, most physicians find this treatment unnecessary. Unless the patient changes the mechanical habits that prompted the condition, the body will return to its former state.

The communication between our brain and our muscles is handled by the muscles' spindles and fibers. The spindles are the sensory unit, while the fibers are the functional unit. Muscle fibers are in themselves divided into intrafusal and extrafusal. The intrafusal fibers are found inside the muscle spindle, which is located in between the extrafusal fibers.

What is interesting about this system is that all of these fibers play a role both in the strengthening of the back muscles as well as in the pain we feel when their parent muscle is out of shape. At the risk of oversimplifying let's see if the following example helps you to understand how this system works.

Let's say you are one of those lucky individuals who looks good even though you are underexercised. In fact it is because of your appearance that you have never thought much about exercise. But today you are asked to pick up a heavy load and carry it for a couple of blocks.

First you think of picking up the object. You have lifted many things before, so your brain has been programmed regarding which muscles to put to work to carry out the action. But the moment you begin to pick up the object, the muscles and brain assess that this time they will require additional strength to carry out the task. Since muscles function as a group, the message is sent out to all the muscles involved in the action, from the deepest to the most superficial layers. The muscles closest to the joint producing the movement will have to work the hardest, while the others may be acting upon other joints to maintain your equilibrium while you are picking up and carrying the object.

As you carry the object your muscles, which are underexercised to begin with, are being taxed to their limit. They become tired and fatigued and send a message to the brain via the sensory nerves saying that they can't take much more of what you are demanding. Now the brain has a dual function. It must do all it can to finish the task it has been asked and it must also increase the strength (contraction) of the muscles to assure that the task is completed. The brain recruits more help from some of its branches of the nervous system glands and organs to come to help and the brain issues a new command. Contract more! This command is sent back to the muscles via the motor end nerves, which are also attached to the muscle spindle. The muscle spindle relays the command to the extrafusal fibers, whose job it is to follow the brain's command.

This is where we start getting into trouble. If the extrafusal fibers of the muscles are out of shape, if they are laden with fat, etc., they will not be able to safely carry out the brain's command. The brain, in its continuous effort to balance out the situation, will then recruit other muscles that might be related to the principal joint involved to help out. Since bad muscle tone is not just found in one muscle but in the entire group, chances are that the new recruits will have the same trouble. The nerves, which are by this time overloaded with complaints, scream out. In a short time an entire area of your back feels as though it's on fire, which the muscles will try to put out by going into spasm, a sudden and final contraction. Why in your back and not in other parts of the body, which are also involved in the action?

Because it is in the back, actually in the entire trunk, that you will find the largest concentration of muscles with extrafusal fibers and it is the extrafusal fibers of the muscles that we target when we exercise. They are the ones that must receive a balanced workload for the development of proper muscle tone.

Extrafusal fibers are in themselves divided into slow twitch and fast twitch fibers. The slow twitch are the ones found in muscles that can respond to work requiring endurance, such as those in our back, stomach and legs. These fibers were not called into action until you attempted to carry the object. The fast twitch fibers are fast acting, or reflex action monitors. They are the ones responsible for fast or impulsive movements, such as getting up quickly from a chair, jumping, starting an action. If you were shoveling snow the fast twitch extrafusal fibers would get you started. If you had to bend down to start the lawnmower the fast twitch extrafusal fibers would pull the arm that pulled the cord. These fibers are also the ones that can pull the muscle into spasm when it isn't ready to pull the cord.

Some anatomists believe that with proper training, a person can change the proportion of these fibers, even though most agree that their number is genetically fixed. Slow twitch fibers, used for endurance, are best trained through aerobic work. They require large amounts of oxygen to keep working, while fast twitch fibers require anaerobic work for strength. This is why proper breathing is necessary while doing any exercise; it serves to improve the all-important oxygen distribution to the muscles of your back and abdomen as you work them, particularly when doing anaerobic exercises.

How much strength is enough for a healthy back? First we must understand how it is measured. Strength is measured by the muscle's ability to move the skeletal structure through the contraction of its fibers. Contrary to popular belief, strength has nothing to do with the size of a muscle; size only indicates the amount of contraction a muscle has been subjected to. If a person's exercise routine has concentrated on contraction by increasing weight resistance (anaerobic exercise), as in weight lifting, a condition called hypertonicity (muscle boundness) develops. Hypertonic muscles exchange suppleness and elasticity for size. Suppleness gives muscles the full range of movement of the joint they move. Therefore, lack of suppleness restricts the range of movement allowed by joint design and promotes stiffness and bad coordination. This is why, in order for any exercise regime to be complete, it must combine *both* anaerobic and aerobic training, for although anaerobic training of long duration does develop a certain degree of aerobic fitness by sheer repetition of the strength-building exercises, it is not enough for proper muscular balance, good muscle tone and prevention of injury.

### Proper Diet for Muscle Function

When a muscle is called to contract, it converts glycogen into lactic acid. This decomposition process, which is reversible, is the muscle's major source of energy. Many factors come together to make this transition a smooth one. Two of the most important ones are a diet that provides a balanced intake of the body's necessary nutrients, and proper breathing.

Water and protein are the most important constituents of muscle tissue. Without adequate protein muscles cannot build new tissues or replace worn-out ones. Proteins contain a series of molecule compounds called amino acids. Approximately twenty-one different amino acids occur in the various forms of proteins. Eight of these are called the essential amino acids. They cannot be manufactured by the body and must therefore be obtained from food. The foods that supply these eight are considered complete proteins, while those that lack them are called incomplete proteins. An adult should take at least one gram of protein daily per kilogram of body weight. Although meat and fish are the most reliable sources of complete protein, other animal sources include egg whites, milk and other dairy products. Vegetarians can receive an adequate amount of proteins from plant sources such as nuts, soybeans and other members of the bean family and by combining them with dairy products. People who engage in strenuous physical activity or work at developing muscle size need larger quantities of protein than the average person.

While complete proteins are needed for the *building* of muscle tissues, muscles get their *energy* from carbohydrates, sugars and starches. The chief sources of carbohydrates are cereals, sugars, vegetables and fruits. While hydrolysis distributes the amino acids to the body's cells as they're needed, it also stores the processed sugar not needed in our muscles and liver in the form of glycogen. When an individual has an unbalanced diet, such as one lacking in protein, the body must use the stored glycogen and convert it for the maintenance of body tissues. Since it is glycogen that is the muscle's source of energy and the prime substance that feeds its contractile mechanism, routing it to other areas depletes and weakens it. This weakening also subjects the muscles and their various forms of attachment, such as tendons and ligaments, to injury. This is another reason why so many people who put themselves on quick weight loss diets end up with more than they bargained for in the way of health problems, among which back pain is common.

### Muscles Need Oxygen

In order to work properly muscles must have oxygen, of which, as we know, the body does not carry a supply. In fact, the body can deplete its oxygen intake in twenty seconds of strenuous activity. Because of the interrelated work of the respiratory, circulatory and nervous systems, oxygen reaches the muscles within seconds, often before actual muscle activity begins. In short, the brain channels oxygen through the circulatory system to the areas it wants to move even before the nerve ends act upon the muscles to initiate movement.

Although breathing is an involuntary act over which we have only some control, it can be assisted by movements which we are able to develop and control. Therefore, the better we know how to breathe the more efficiently our muscles will function. Proper breathing habits, as we will see in Section Two, are easy to develop and crucial to the mechanical function of the muscles. Correct breathing also contributes to the rehabilitation of injured muscles and, when it's combined with relaxation techniques, the alleviation of pain.

### Nerves and Muscles

Body movement occurs through the cooperation of the central nervous system, its branches and the interpolation of these branches in our muscles. Before we move we think movement. The pictured action is then sent from the brain to the muscles designated to carry it out. Once the action starts, the muscles will keep feeding the brain information about the environmental conditions, the obstacles faced and what is needed to overcome those obstacles as movement develops, continues or stops.

Our nervous system runs through practically every part of our back through branches of nerve roots that are connected to the vertebrae, the fibrous shell of the discs, ligaments and the muscles that provide movement and flexibility. There are thirty-one pair of spinal nerves which exit from the different curves of the spine. One branch covers the muscles and skin of the back, while the other branch covers the muscles and skin on the side and front of the body.

As we've seen, there are five curves in the spine. The nerves emanating from the cervical or neck area (eight pair) and the lumbar curve (five pair) are those most prone to injury because of the wide range of movement possible in these curves. The main cervical nerves branch out to cover the shoulders and arms. The spinal cord ends at the level of the first lumbar vertebra, where it divides into main nerves. These nerves exit from the lumbar vertebrae and upper sacral vertebrae, then join again to form the sciatic nerves, which run down the backs of the legs.

Although there are several small muscles around the cervical vertebrae, most movement in this area is controlled by the trapezius muscle. Shaped like a kite, it covers the largest portion of the back by running from the neck to the lower back (the tail of the kite), and from shoulder to shoulder above the shoulder blades, the movement of which it controls. Trouble in any of the cervical vertebrae, their nerves or muscles can be felt in a variety of ways. The ones to be most aware of are tingling sensations, numbness, stiffness and impaired movement of the arms.

When the back muscles, especially the trapezius, are out of tone, a simple movement such as reaching for an object on a high shelf or even closing the blinds can cause a sudden burst of pain that feels as though it's coming from the neck, even though in actuality there is nothing wrong with any of the cervical vertebrae.

One of the main reasons that pain due to muscle spasm is not always felt at its point of origin is because our bodies have numerous layers of muscles. Each muscle is connected to a series of sensory and motor end nerves that branch out from nerve fibers. These in turn come from main nerves that unite and then subdivide before entering the spinal cord. Back pain can result from an unfavorable sensation picked up by a nerve from a facet joint, from a disc that is pressing on it, from a ligament or, as in the majority of cases, from a nerve in one of the many muscles covering the back.

## MUSCLE TONE

Keeping your back healthy and functioning properly is synonomous with keeping its muscles in good tone. Muscle tone is measured by the time it takes a person's muscles to reach a resting state after activity, and by the amount of tension left in them when at rest. Degree of muscle tone depends on the amount of balanced work, specifically contraction and extension, that a muscle or group of muscles has been subjected to. Exercise is the only known method to increase and maintain good muscle tone.

Because all muscles respond to the same method of conditioning, an individual study of the muscles of the back is not necessary for proper maintenance. Their interrelated characteristics make it possible for them to benefit from unilateral conditioning. It is important to remember that muscles in good condition need *constant* care. People who only exercise sporadically are as prone to back injury as those who never exercise.

How much exercise is enough?

Research studies show that thirty minutes of aerobic exercise (i.e., jogging, jumping rope, swimming, bicycling, etc.) balanced with anaerobic or strength-building exercise (i.e., curls, push-ups, etc.) done three times a week is sufficient for the average person to maintain proper muscle tone and low body fat. The flexibility test on page 80 can also help to determine the areas of muscle weakness and tightness which should be worked on. If you are underexercised, you will have to start out more slowly than the recommended thirty minute period—short periods of exercise, alternated with periods of resting and stretching is a sensible way to begin a fitness program. The exercises in this book are designed to get you started if you're underexercised, or if you're resuming exercise after a back injury.

One can also have medically-supervised tests taken that specifically determine a person's present muscular condition, cardiovascular fitness and amount of body fat. The result of such tests are then used by experts to devise an exercise program tailored to your state of fitness. Hospitals and other medical facilities as well as some private institutions with a sports medicine department offer such examinations, as do most YMCAs. Needless to say, these examinations are costly.

### The Overload Principle

The safest way to strengthen muscles is by putting them through gradually intensified workouts over a period of time. Muscles must be worked at progressively repetitive intervals, each of which must surpass the degree of intensity reached at the previous interval. This is called the Overload Principle. As most theories go, it has a good and a bad side. The positive effects of utilizing the Overload Principle are that it gets your back into shape, it makes you look better, walk better, feel better, and in general makes you a more physically fit person.

The negative effect of the Overload Principle is that it is reversible; this means that using it will get you into shape, but it can also result in your getting out of shape faster. This is seen primarily in people who exercise excessively or who exercise for cosmetic reasons only (which can lead to extremes), rather than for proper maintenance of their bodies and health.

The way in which we can get out of shape fast is closely related to back problems, especially in individuals who have always been in top shape and would seem to be the least likely candidates for back problems. This is how it happens:

The tone of your muscles largely depends on the type of exercise you subject them to. For instance, if you do free hand exercises (without weights) such as calisthenics or dance chances are that your muscles will be more lean, longer-looking and will have the necessary strength for moderate to heavy, although not strenuous, activity. Your muscle fibers will be strong, but not bulky. If you do aerobic exercises you can endure more vigorous physical activity for longer periods of time, but your muscles will tend to have less elasticity. Running, especially, is one aerobic exercise that tends to tighten the major muscle groups of the hips, thighs, and legs. If you exercise exclusively with weights and fail to balance your work out with the exercises that will improve cardiovascular system and elasticity and flexibility of the muscles, your muscle fibers will grow thicker.

Now, let's say that you are someone who has worked out consistently week after week, but for some reason you must stop because of a vacation, illness, schedule conflict or whatever. The fibers in your muscles, which have been kept strengthened and have been subjected to periodic tension, will relax and become thinner. Since you are not exercising you are not burning as many calories, though you are probably eating the same amount of food or more. The extra calories you consume deposit themselves in the pockets that have formed between the now thinner muscle fibers. The bigger the fibers once were, they sooner they will thin out and the larger the pockets will be that are formed. Before you know it your formerly lean muscle has become fat at an alarming rate. Its tone has decreased. Unaware of this, you go back to your exercise schedule and start where you left off, probably exercising even harder, thinking that you will make up for lost time. And boom! Your back, which thinks you're still on vacation, goes out on you.

The other way in which the Overload Principle reverses itself has to do with age. As we get older, we become less concerned with having the trimmest or most muscular body on the block. Our lives change, priorities are reestablished and unlimited periods of time for workouts become a thing of the past. In addition our metabolic rate, which is the body's calorie-burning mechanism, decreases, while too often our appetite does not. We burn fewer calories due to less exercise while we continue to take in the same amount as before. The muscle fibers which were enlarged through the "pumping iron" years become thinner and develop pockets between them, where the extra calories find comfortable retirement. This is why a muscularly overdeveloped person runs the risk of becoming much flabbier in later years than his normally fit counterpart. This is seen more frequently in men because men's hormonal composition allows their muscle fibers to enlarge more and faster, although women may also encounter the same problem to a lesser degree.

### Muscle Sprains or Strains

The confusion between sprains and strains arises from the similarity of their sound. A sprain applies to ligaments that have been overstretched (pulled beyond their capabilities) or torn from the bones they are connected to. Not all ligaments have the same amount of elasticity. The most nonelastic ones can be forcibly stretched until they are permanently lengthened and thus become inefficient. In the spine we find more elastic ligaments than in other sections of the body. A prime example is the Ligament Flava, which runs the length of the spine. With continuous stretching this ligament can lose its elasticity and is unable to return to its normal size. A common example of this is seen in people with a round or hunched back, and is often due to sitting for long periods of time hunched over a desk, typewriter, etc.

While ligaments join bones together, tendons are the fibrous bands that attach muscles to the bone. Because they have more elastic properties than ligaments, they can resist stretching to a larger degree. If stretched too much they can tear at the junction of either muscle or bone or they can become wrenched or strained. A prime example is the Achilles tendon which can easily become strained (tendonitis) when it isn't properly stretched before and after jogging or aerobic dancing.

### Trigger Points

Trigger points are painful muscular conditions usually felt on the neck, shoulders, or upper back areas and can be caused by sprains or strains. They can also be the result of postural deviations, such as sleeping with the neck crooked, and are characterized by localized areas in the skin which, when pressed on, can shoot out agonizing pain in several directions. Doctors frequently relieve the pain caused by trigger points by injecting the area with a local anesthetic. Although relief is felt immediately after an injection, it may take more than one shot over a period of time to eradicate the pain permanently.

### Muscle Spasm

Muscle spasm is an involuntary contraction by a muscle or group of muscles that has been signaled by the central nervous system to respond to a command. A spasm results when the command taxes one, all or a combination of muscles. This sudden contraction can produce a series of chain reactions. As the muscle contracts, the increased pulling force it exerts can cause tears in the muscle fibers and in the tendons that connect the muscle to the bones; it can render the muscle totally immobile through the depletion of oxygen and the accumulation of lactic acid, which will delay an easing of tension; it can decrease the muscle's ability to respond to further command (irritability); it can bring total fatigue to the muscle. Even muscles that have a fairly good degree of tone can, in reaction to an unfavorable action, go into spasm, but conditioned muscles will return to a resting state much faster than muscles that are out of shape.

Still, this is not the whole story of what can bring about muscle spasm, since many times it is not solely mechanical in origin. Muscle spasm can also result from changes and adjustments induced by the central nervous system, which sends out messages to its main branches and their sensory subdivisions. This wide communication network, which is responsible for all bodily functions, is also responsible for the body's perception, assimilation and reflex action to any outside stimuli. Whenever we are exposed to situations that demand more concentration or alertness, or involve new or increased physical activity, our body goes through chemical reactions in preparation for those changes. This is especially true of times when we take on physical work that is not part of our regular routine.

As an example of these chemical changes and how they relate to muscle spasm and back pain, let's take a hypothetical situation, such as the painting of a room, which has placed many amateur decorators in bed with roller in hand and pain, instead of paint, dripping down their backs.

Even before the paint is poured the central nervous system has been readying itself for the job from the moment you thought about it. If you have painted a room before, your brain has stored knowledge of what was done and will feed the information to your muscles as needed. In this case the chemical changes and adjustments made will be less intense than if you've never painted before. But let's assume that this is your first time. The moment you pick up the roller your central nervous system will increase your heart rate, therefore, your blood supply. It will also increase the distribution of sugar and fats to produce more fuel and will increase muscle tension to prepare the body for the action. If your muscles lack tone, which means they already have tensed fibers, you won't be able to perform the job as smoothly and your body will use more energy than if you were in good shape. The more energy required, the more tension must be placed on the muscles. And just as you are reaching up to paint the ceiling the muscles of the back and the shoulders stretch beyond what their present state of conditioning will allow. This is when the muscles revolt, shooting pain up your back. Thus, an action that started in your head was channeled to your muscles, which returned the signal back to your brain in a painful state. The signal was then transmitted back to the muscles by the brain in the form of spasm.

The above example also illustrates why warming up before beginning any exercise routine, including running, is of the utmost importance, for when the muscles are not ready to move into action, they can and often will revolt in the form of a spasm.

# CAUSES OF BACK PAIN

There are numerous causes of back pain and, to complicate matters further, many of the different causes are so closely interrelated that it is often difficult for a doctor to give an accurate diagnosis without some careful examination. This is one reason why many orthopedists will refer their back patients to other physicians who are known as "back doctors." Although it is certainly beneficial to consult more than one doctor, it can add to a patient's confusion, if only because doctors quite typically describe any one condition in a variety of ways.

Of all the things that can cause back pain, the *least* common cause involves pathological disorders. More often it's brought about by degenerative disorders, traumatic disorders, metabolic disorders, mechanical disorders and emotional disorders. And although some pathological causes of back pain are mechanically related, most are strictly mechanical or of a skeletal or muscular nature, compounded by emotional disorders. Before discussing the other more common causes, let's take a look at some of the most common pathological disorders that can bring about back pain.

## PATHOLOGICAL CAUSES

Pathological causes of back pain can be due to tumors, kidney stones or kidney infections, hip disease, different forms of arthritis, prostate problems in men and uterine tumors in women. They can also be mechanical in origin, or related to mechanical conditions such as scoliosis (lateral deviation of the spine) which, if left unattended throughout a person's formative or early adult years, can worsen, possibly causing arthritic complications.

### Osteoarthritis
Osteoarthritis is a degenerative disorder that appears in middle age and is considered a rheumatic condition. It is characterized by the disintegration of the cartilage that lines the facet joints of the vertebrae. Depending on whether the degeneration is total (in advanced cases) or partial, the disorder stems from the bones of the two adjoining vertebrae grinding

against each other, producing tremendous pain. In total disintegration, entrapment of the nerves (which is commonly referred to as a "pinched nerve") can make this condition even more painful.

Osteoarthritis is not limited to the spine; it may also occur in the knees, ankles and hips. Although it is a very common form of arthritis, it is seen more frequently in people who are overweight and/or those who have a history of it in the family. People under fifty seldom develop this condition, although it is seen in athletes who have suffered joint sprains and the like during their active years. I must note that during one of my interviews with a physician who specializes in treating senior citizens, I mentioned my adoptive grandmother who, at age ninety-six, can give Ginger Rogers a run for her money, even though she's had a hip fracture. I also mentioned that she's never had any arthritic problem. The doctor asked me if she exercised. I told him that for the last thirty years she has watched her diet, stays slim and goes to a dancing club three times a week. She's even won some dancing trophies! He confirmed that her good health and exercise habits have freed her from arthritic pain, a lesson from which we all can learn.

### Spondylosis

This is another degenerative condition which causes changes in the intervertebral disc. The disc can be totally absorbed as a result of repeated stress and strain to its vertebrae throughout a person's life. It is seen mostly in the cervical area, but when it occurs in the lumbar vertebrae it can cause a complete collapse of this area, which will interfere with a person's mobility. When spondylosis combines with osteoarthritis it is called degenerative hypertrophic spondylitis. The following suggestions have been found to be quite successful in the treatment of this, as in most other arthritic conditions: loss of weight to reduce pressure on the joints, avoidance of any kind of activity that produces extra pressure on the joints, such as lifting objects or heavy housework, exercise that prevents atrophy of major muscles in the legs and trunk, and stretching exercises that induce flexibility in the joints (in Section Two there is a whole group of stretching exercises that promote flexibility).

### Herniated Disc (Slipped Disc)

When back pain hits, most people immediately think it's due to a slipped disc without knowing what it means. Later on in the section on discs you will learn not only that discs cannot "slip," but that problems with vertebral discs are rare. If you do have a herniated or slipped disc, that means that the center of the disc (nucleus pulposus), which is encased by a fibrous shell, has undergone certain degenerative changes which could cause some or all of its contents to pour out through an opening of that shell. The direction in which this spillage flows (it usually flows toward the back of the vertebrae where the spinal canal is located), can determine the type of pain it can cause. The pain would be felt down the leg if the herniated disc was pressing on a nerve, such as the sciatic nerve. Discs are usually herniated in the two areas of the spine where there is the most mobility, that is, in the cervical and the lumbar areas. But it is in the latter, especially between the two lowest lumbar vertebrae and the first sacral vertebra, that this condition is found, where most of the major nerves are found that travel to the lower limbs. This is why pain is felt in the legs. The pain will be localized according to the nerve that is pinched, which makes identification and diagnosis easier for your physician.

Herniated discs in children, an even rarer occurrence, have been diagnosed as due to a condition called autoimmune disease, which is an allergic chemical reaction children may develop to cells in their own bodies. This reaction will cause degenerative changes, of which a herniated disc is one. I must emphasize that this condition is extremely rare and, unfortunately, very little is known about it.

Although a disc can herniate due to an accident, herniation by degeneration seldom occurs in people who have kept their muscles in good tone through regular exercise and their weight down through proper nutrition.

### Spinal Stenosis

This is another degenerative disease which is commonly found in people over the age of seventy. It results from a combination of spondylosis in the discs and osteoarthritis in the facet joints. Sometimes bony growths that come out of the facet joints lodge themselves in the spinal canal, pressing nerves or even preventing nerves from exiting. Total degeneration of the discs is also possible, in which case the nerves of the area become totally entrapped by the pressure of both vertebrae and the further narrowing of the space from which spinal nerves exit, causing tremendous pain. Most of the Tension Relief Exercises listed in the second section will give some relief for this if pain is not too acute. These exercises, especially those in which I recommend forward bending of the trunk, will increase the spaces between the lumbar vertebrae and relieve some of the pressure on the nerve.

## METABOLIC DISORDERS

### Osteoporosis

Osteoporosis is a bone disease which, for the most part, occurs in later years. Its victims are usually women who have gone through meno-pause. It is not limited to the bones of the spine, but can affect all of the bones of the skeleton. It is characterized by the bones becoming unusually thin, making them prone to injury and fracture. It is believed that the best way to avoid osteoporosis is to stay active, exercise regularly and eat a balanced diet that includes calcium as well as vitamin D. In some women estrogen is administered which, although it cannot rebuild lost bone, can help prevent future loss and even offer pain relief. Swimming and walking are excellent exercise for those who suffer from osteoporosis.

## TRAUMATIC DISORDERS

Most traumatic disorders are those caused by an external force, such as an accident. It is important to note that accidents that involve fractures of the spine are rare. Nevertheless the most common affecting this area are:

### Spondylolysis
This condition exists when a vertebra, for reasons not really known, weakens and a portion of its vertebral arch cracks or breaks, sometimes separating it from the vertebral body. This is usually seen in the lumbar area and produces intermittent pain. It could be the result of a fracture suffered during childhood that was not detected or did not heal properly. In later years, as continued stress is applied, it may resurface. It is also believed that this condition might be genetically influenced. In some cases the breaking of the vertebral arch will cause the vertebral body to slip forward. When this happens the condition is known as spondylolisthesis.

### Spondylolisthesis
As mentioned above, it is the result of a vertebra that has slipped away from the adjoining ones due to either a genetic weakening of the vertebrae or fracture. This condition is seen quite frequently in athletes whose profession requires them to perform movements where they must bend backward repeatedly, such as swimmers who specialize in the butterfly stroke, gymnasts, football players and pole vaulters.

### Fracture of the Transverse Process
This is also common in athletes. It can be caused by a forceful pull of muscles which can crack or break the transverse or the spinous process of a vertebra. Usually rest will take care of the condition unless spondylo-listhesis occurs. If it does, surgery may be required, after which the patient can resume normal activity after recovery.

### Subluxated Facet

This is the most common cause of back pain when you have been doing some physical activity like shoveling snow or moving a heavy object and all of a sudden can't straighten up. The little facet joints that connect the vertabrae have come out of alignment and cause tremendous pain because either the bones have been allowed to rub together, a nerve is pressed, a ligament is stretched or a muscle is pulled. Subluxated facets respond to manipulation techniques. They are the ones that make those cracking sounds when your back is being put back into proper alignment.

## MECHANICAL DISORDERS

Body mechanics are determined by the manner in which muscles move the skeletal structure. Therefore when we speak of mechanical disorders of the back we are talking about a series of malfunctions, most of which are caused by abnormalities of the spine, ligament strain, muscular spasm and emotional stress. These problems can be further compounded by skeletal misalignment, bad posture, bad body mechanics and lack of muscular tone.

### Causes of Mechanical Disorders:

*1. Structural abnormalities of the spine.* "If you took one hundred people off the street that have never had back pain and X-rayed their backs you would probably find twenty or thirty percent of them with some abnormality," says Dr. Hamilton. Research studies have shown that genetics influence our backs. It is not difficult, for instance, to find people who have one or two extra vertebrae in their coccyx or tail bone, just like their mother had. Others might have one less lumbar vertebra and one additional sacral vertebra. Many people have extreme lordosis (swaybacks), which can become increasingly accented by poor mechanical habits, bad posture, age and being overweight. Many of them will never experience any trouble because of it but it is still like carrying a bomb that could go off at any moment. Scoliosis, a sideward deviation of the spine, is often found among members of one family.

In some cases of spinal abnormalities, as in some cases of herniated discs, surgery is the only solution, after which medically supervised exercise and rehabilitation treatment is the best therapy for resumption of normal activity. Again, abnormalities are at the bottom of the list of causes of back pain.

*2. Ligament strain.* The vertebrae of the spine are joined together by a series of ligaments. They act as a part of the mechanism that supports and allows for the flexibility of the spine. When the muscles of the trunk are weak, ligaments tend to work beyond their capability to compensate for the muscle's strength deficiency. As a result the ligaments can become strained, causing pain. They may also become injured if the structures to which they are attached, such as vertebrae, are themselves in poor condition. First bed rest, then gradual exercise for muscle strengthening are the best cure.

When a ligament has been severely strained recovery could take between six and twelve weeks. Immobilization of the affected area is the usual principle of therapy. During acute pain after an injury the best thing to do is to apply something cold, such as an ice bag or cold water bottle. This will reduce circulation and thus swelling, but after the third or fourth day, heat is the recommended treatment to improve circulation, avoid further stiffness and the possibility of muscle spasm.

*3. Muscular spasm.* Dr. Nagler, whose work in back care and rehabilitation has set precedents in the field, has said that among the causes of back pain, muscle spasm is at the top of the list. Muscle spasms are mainly caused by poor muscle tone due to incorrect or no exercise. Although it is rather difficult to separate back-related problems due to muscular spasms from those caused by other mechanical and psychological reasons, there are several specific muscular conditions which often contribute to back pain, as discussed in the section on muscles. If you are recovering from muscular spasm, see Section Two for different methods of muscular strengthening, relaxation and rehabilitation.

*4. Emotional Stress.* Last and certainly not least in the causes of back pain is emotional stress. Many doctors believe it is the number one cause. But emotional stress is not necessarily bad for you. In fact, we need stress in order to reach new challenges as well as surpass previous ones. Studies have shown that people produce better under some stress than under none at all. It is also known that there is very little difference in the chemical and hormonal reactions that our bodies produce from positive stress such as that created by elation, love, laughter, recognition, etc., and that created by frustration, depression, fear, anxiety, etc. Furthermore it is widely accepted that it is the way in which we view stressful situations that largely determines our reactions to them.

While it is a physiological fact that all emotional stress begins in the mind, why is it that our backs are the place where all of it seems to express itself? Although that may seem to be the case, stress, just like body fat, may be localized in some areas more than others, but it *is* manifested in all parts of the body.

In the October 1982 issue of *Psychology Today*, a survey was taken in which the majority of people who responded said they felt that stress was the number one cause of personal unhappiness and lack of well-being in their lives. The polled readers agreed that "Things in life that make you nervous, angry or unhappy" should be eliminated. This, of course, is not possible, for if it were we could never drive in rush hour traffic, hold down a responsible job or have arguments with our spouses. We can't and don't live our lives in closets, which would supposedly be stress-free environments. What, then, is the alternative? The secret to physical well-being lies not in avoiding stress, which is always around us and unavoidable, but in understanding it, coping with it, even reaping benefits from it, but not being negatively controlled by it.

Although the psychology of emotional stress is well beyond the scope of this book, two important facts that relate to stress and our backs do come to mind: one, because of the array of nerves and muscles that cover our backs, the tension that accompanies all stressful situations is felt in this area more than in any other part of the body; and two, medical science has proven beyond a doubt that exercise is the most effective form of alleviating stress, while proper nutrition is the second.

What most doctors, unfortunately, do not tell their patients is how to use exercise to relieve stress. They just say, "Your back hurts because you are out of shape and overweight. You are nervous and tense. Go out and exercise. Take up jogging, lose some weight." So people attempt to do just that. They go out and exercise and while exercising they are still thinking and worrying about all the problems they have. They are not thinking about the exercise they are doing. Actually, and this is an opinion I have developed from seeing hundreds of people exercise, they are getting more tense and receiving little or no benefit from their physical struggles. In fact, they are running a bigger risk of injuring themselves than if they just stayed home and did nothing. In order to relax one's muscles one must coordinate the mind and the body. In order to benefit from exercise one must do the same.

A muscle, in order to be stretched, must be given time to relax. This process involves the circulatory, respiratory and nervous systems, as well as the range of mobility of the body's joints and levers. It must all be coordinated—carefully. Otherwise it is a waste of time. The same goes for exercises geared to relax the mind. You can't just sit quietly in a corner, hoping that because you are not moving you are going to relax. You must concentrate on relaxing. Point and degree of concentration are achieved, just as good muscle tone is, through practice.

### How Stress-induced Muscle Tension Causes Back Pain
Modern psychology has shown that the control of stress, which is

necessary to control muscular tension, depends on the proportional balance between the two sub-branches of the nervous system, the sympathetic and parasympathetic. Much of what is known today about stress is taken from studies done by Dr. Walter Bradford Cannon and Dr. Hans Selye, who coined the term "stress" in the 1930s. Dr. Selye described the sympathetic system as the manner in which the body responds to anything perceived as a possible threat—it is the body's alert system, which triggers the "fight or flight" response.

Let's look at a hypothetical situation to see how the sympathetic system works: You smell smoke in your house, then you spot the fire. The emotional stress the situation triggers moves the sympathetic system into action which, in turn, triggers glandular secretion in the endocrine glands. Adrenaline is poured into the body; your heart beat and blood pressure increase; the stomach slows down the digestive process. The muscles of the trunk, the most affected area, go into a state of contraction and tension. Your body is in a heightened state of alert which you will respond to either by running (flight) or getting water or an extinguisher (fight). All of these reactions have been activated by the sympathetic system within seconds of your smelling smoke. Furthermore, the sympathetic system helped to activate your mental faculties by increasing the brain's level of concentration.

The parasympathetic system oversees the maintenance of the body's organs. Its function is to cool the body down and return it to a resting state after arousal—it is the inhibiting force of the nervous system. These two systems must work together to maintain an overall balance of the vital organs they affect. In Dr. Phil Nuernberger's book, *Freedom from Stress—A Holistic Approach* (Himalayan International Institute) he writes, "By arbitrarily (but not necessarily consciously) paying attention to certain cues and not to other cues in the world, we, in a very real sense, program what we want our experiences in life to be." Often when the results don't match up with our initial expectations in any given situation, we respond with stress.

To better understand how stress affects the body, in particular the back, let's return to the example of the fire and combine it with another situation.

Let's assume that you were that person who smelled smoke and discovered the fire, and your body underwent the various physical and chemical changes we've discussed. It is three years later and you've just come home from a hard day at the office. Physically your body is not in the best condition possible—it is tired and, to some degree, tense. You find that that evening you have to perform some strenuous physical task, like moving a heavy object or maybe you have to shovel snow. Before you carry out the task let's say that you've come across something that reminds you of that earlier fire—maybe you watched the news or read the paper and learned of a similar incident. What happens? Your sympathetic system is activated by your mental process of thinking of the fire—a threat is perceived, regardless that it happened some time ago. Your brain immediately brings out the file that stored the information about the fire and your body again undergoes some or all of the chemical changes it originally experienced, except for one important difference—your sympathetic system of arousal has been activated but there is no need for it to move you into action—the flight or fight response is not triggered. Although your body is undergoing chemical changes, this time there is no physical release for the adrenaline and other glandular substances which are secreted. And although your mind may quickly forget about the fire, it will take time for that extra tension in your muscles to dissipate. Now let's say you're ready to perform that physical task that awaits you. Because of the added tension, you begin with reduced muscular elasticity and flexibility. You may be as tight as a rope. If you are, as you bend down and pull the muscles into action, chances are the muscles will go into spasm.

There is very little that can influence our reaching a relaxed state before, during and after exercise as can the combination of proper breathing, a positive mental attitude and concentration while exercising and stretching the muscles.

All of the stretching exercises that you will find in Section Two are devised with you and your back in mind. Even if you hate these exercises, which many people do, you will find these stretches of tremendous value in alleviating muscular and nervous tension.

Although a back free of pain cannot exist without proper exercise, this in turn cannot be achieved without the interaction of the mind, the nervous system and the positive attitude of your desire. If you make a conscious effort to combine these things, a back free of pain can be yours.

## MISCELLANEOUS CAUSES OF BACK PAIN

As if there weren't enough reasons for back pain, it can also develop through self-infliction or autosuggestion. Some doctors call it hysteria while others call it hypochrondia. I recently spoke with a physician who told me about a patient who had all the classic symptoms of back pain, along with some very specific symptoms that had been described in a television special which the doctor had seen as well. Oddly enough, in talking with other doctors, I found that they, too, had had similar experiences with some of their patients who developed "symptoms" after reading or hearing about them. This manifestation of back pain could be thought of as back pain through suggestion.

Throughout this decade health and fitness are topics which have received more media coverage than ever before. This has been of great benefit in making us aware of the importance of taking care of ourselves. But programs focusing on health hazards and rare disorders can influence some people tremendously, and not for the better.

Take, for example, someone who has had a common case of lower back pain, but has been under tremendous emotional stress as well. This person may have just seen a television special about heart attacks, cancer, strokes, what have you. For some people, the stress is enough to trigger a reaction so that the lower back pain symptoms become more complex and painful, possibly by their taking on some of the symptoms they have just seen or read about. For treatment of such patients, medical science often has to take a Sherlock Holmes approach and must try to sort out the real from the unreal. Whether it's hypochondria, psychosomatic symptoms, mental stress or something else, the reality remains that the pain that is triggered really does hurt, even if there's no physical cause.

Another common example of how back pain can get worse through suggestion is by listening to other people's experiences with back trouble. Imagine that you get up one Monday morning feeling stiff and your back hurts a little. Never mind that during the weekend you had your first game of touch football in twenty years or you went dancing for the first time since Elvis Presley returned from boot camp. You notice that your walk is different; you can't even stand up straight. Something doesn't feel quite right. You feel as though needles were pricking you all over. It even hurts to pick up the phone and call the office to say you won't be in. You talk to one of your co-workers, who tells you about someone who had similar back pain. That person has been in bed for six months. You panic! You hurt even more . . . This is another reason why it's important to stay as relaxed as possible when back pain strikes—and try not to pay too much attention to anyone else's back problems that you might hear about. Remember, too, if your doctor doesn't see a reason to be alarmed, neither should you.

# ARE YOU A BACK PAIN CANDIDATE?

As previously stated, back pain can be caused by a number of things, although muscular problems and stress are the main causes. What are the factors that contribute to muscular problems? Taking a look at those factors can be of great help in understanding the source of the pain. The following questionnaire lists common contributors to back pain and can help determine whether or not you are a likely candidate for it. If you are presently experiencing difficulties, the questions may point out a possible cause of your present condition.

1. Do you sleep on a firm mattress?
2. Do you sleep on your back?
3. Do you sleep by an air conditioner or an open window?
4. Do you have the type of job that requires travel and doesn't allow you to sleep on your own mattress regularly?
5. Do you sleep using a lot of pillows?
6. Do you drive long distances frequently?
7. Does your car seat have a lower back support?
8. Do you stretch your legs out to reach the pedals or do you slouch when you drive?
9. Do you carry a wallet in your back pocket?
10. Do you sit a lot throughout the day?
11. When you sit are your knees at hip level or higher?
12. Do you make a point of standing and limbering up every couple of hours?
13. Do you stand a lot throughout the day?
14. Do you maintain the same standing position for long periods?
15. Do you wear boots or high-heeled shoes frequently?
16. If you watch television for long periods of time, do you face it straight ahead while sitting in a comfortable chair or do you face it sideways while lying on a couch?

17. Are you in the habit of carrying a shoulder bag?
18. If so, do you always carry it on the same side?
19. Do you take care of small children?
20. Have you ever had problems with your kidneys?
21. Do you suffer from constipation?
22. Have you ever had a history of rectal bleeding?
23. Do you have prostate problems?
24. Have you recently engaged in a sexual relationship with a new partner?
25. Are you undergoing menopause?
26. Do you suffer from severe menstrual cramps?
27. Have you experienced any major changes in your life recently?
28. Are you planning to make any major changes in the near future?
29. Are you on a quick weight-loss diet?
30. Are you an exercise buff who has recently taken a long vacation during which you did not exercise?
31. Have you recently started to jog, but haven't exercised for a long time before doing so?

Even if you answered no to all of the previous questions, there are still countless hidden reasons that could be the cause of a present or future case of back pain.

Physicians use the results of certain flexibility tests to help determine what could be the cause of back pain. The tests target abdominal strength and back strength as well as flexibility of the back, hips and legs. Give yourself the following tests to discover if you are a likely candidate for back pain. Of course if you are presently in pain, giving yourself this test is not only unnecessary, but it could aggravate your present condition.

*Test #1.* First lie down on the floor with your legs straight in front of you. Can you roll up into a sitting position without lifting your legs off the floor as your torso comes up?

*Test #2.* Can you lift both legs off the floor and hold them for ten counts? If you try this and feel strain in your back, don't lower your legs quickly, but bend them at the knees instead and place your feet on the floor. Stay in that position for a few minutes.

*Test #3.* Lying on your stomach with fingers laced behind your neck, can you lift your torso off the floor without lifting your legs and hold the position for ten counts?

*Test #4.* While standing with feet parallel about six inches apart, can you bend down and touch your toes? If not, can you get as far as your ankles?

Although these tests, which are given by many physicians to back patients, are designed to determine a person's strength as well as flexibility, they are not full proof in determining your chances of back pain. But they are about the best indicators there are without a complete examination. One thing they will prove, however, is that if you can't successfully carry out these tests, or even one of them, you are underexercised. And that is tantamount to being a prime candidate for back pain.

This last questionnaire is directed to expectant and new mothers:

1. Did you have a regular exercise schedule before pregnancy?
2. Are you exercising regularly during pregnancy?
3. Have you gained more than ten pounds during pregnancy in excess of what your doctor has advised?
4. Have you suffered from hemorrhoids during pregnancy?
5. Did you start to exercise as soon after delivery as was recommended by your doctor?

If you had difficulty completing the test, the exercises in the next section will be of much help in gradually toning your muscles and strengthening your back. Remember that if you are experiencing back trouble as you read this, do not start the rehabilitative exercises until your doctor tells you it is safe to do so.

# SECTION

2

# YOU, YOUR BACK
# AND EXERCISE

If you have a back problem and your doctor has told you it's because of lack of exercise, you are not alone. Despite the fitness craze that has taken over the country in the past few years, the fact remains that the vast majority of our population is still overfed and underexercised. As I mentioned earlier, three out of every five adults will know how painfully stubborn their backs can be at least once in their lifetime. True, there are a lot of people who don't exercise and haven't yet had back trouble, but chances are their luck will change and they'll join that percentage of people who do have it.

Why are so many of us reluctant to stay on—or start—a regular exercise program? The truth is, even among those of us who do exercise regularly, that it's considered a bore. In previous times, before our lives were made easy with every imaginable gadget and appliance, exercise wasn't necessary—our bodies were worked out in the course of the day, whether it was through washing clothes by hand or working in the fields. Today, of course, it takes a concerted effort for us to exercise our bodies as much as they needed it. I have spent my entire life exercising and teaching others how to exercise. And even I concede that at times it *is* boring, although I try to make my classes as enjoyable as possible.

And so what is the solution to this modern dilemma? The secret to exercise as part of a daily routine lies in our ability to do one of three things: 1) find a way to make it fun, which is not always possible; 2) find a way to make it convenient to your schedule, which is just a little more possible; or 3) make it into an experience that is both relaxing and invigorating. This is the most likely angle to pursue since it has direct payoffs, but it takes a certain amount of guidance and planning. The one thing that you must *never* do in regard to exercise is to put it off for as long as you can, such as waiting until your doctor tells you have a weak back, or until a friend or spouse tells you you're getting flabby.

## HOW TO MAKE BACK EXERCISES WORK FOR YOU

1. It is recommended that you do exercises in this section, especially the Daily Rehab Conditioners, in the morning, about half an hour after waking up and in the evening, at least two hours before or after a meal. Exercise in the morning is beneficial because your muscles are still very relaxed after sleep. A work-out at this time will also increase your metabolic rate for the next five or six hours, helping your body to burn calories more quickly. Exercise in the evening also has its benefits because it serves to release any tension that may have been built up during the day. It also will not make you hungry.

2. Choose a place that is free from distraction or noise. The exercises do not take much room so most any place will do. Take the phone off the hook!

3. Exercise on a rug or thin exercise mat—don't use a heavily cushioned one.

4. If your time is limited and you can't set aside fifteen or twenty minutes, just do the Tension Release Exercises instead of the Daily Rehab routine. It will be a waste of your time to try to rush through them all.

5. If you have a stereo select some soothing music to exercise to.

6. Spend a few seconds practicing the breathing exercises in the following chapter. They will help you clear your mind of any distractions or negative thoughts, and the increased oxygen intake will invigorate you and add to your muscle tone.

There are actually two advantages to exercise when you must do it after back trouble. One is that you must be careful not to work your muscles too hard, or exert yourself too much; you must do them gradually, but frequently. In fact, exercises for rehabilitation of the back must be done every day, although you'll find that they are not strenuous. The other advantage is that the amount of time you spend on exercises for your back averages to about fifteen minutes a day, much less than that required in a regular exercise program. So give your back a good break. Don't just leaf through the exercises. You have come this far. I promise you will find them easy to do and not time consuming. And more important, they will make your entire body, not just your back, feel so good that you will realize that the few minutes spent each day will be well worth the effort for a pain-free back.

## EXERCISING UP WITH THE JONESES

Even if two months ago you were an All-American linebacker, the moment your back "touched down" you joined the ranks of those of us who wait in line for tickets. Start slowly and easily. Don't push it! There is a special section of stretching exercises at the end of this chapter for athletes with back injuries.

To the rest of us ticket buyers I have a few more words of advice . . . Regardless of the attention that physical fitness has received in the last two decades, the overwhelming majority of people still know little about the proper way to stay fit. And even though exercise by any means is better than none, taking a good honest look at our capabilities and limitations is the first safety prerequisite for smart exercising. Too many people will go to a gym, for instance, and see someone with a beautifully developed body doing some kind of exercise. They will think that perhaps they should try it, too, without giving any thought to the fact that this person has gone through great pains and many stages to get his or her body to where it is. So, think smart before you embark on those leg raises on the slant bar or the sit-ups with the ten-pound weights hanging around your neck.

Remember, too, that proper stretching of your muscles before and after each workout is of optimum importance. Stretching contributes to the muscle's flexibility and its general tone. In this book you will find several different stretch routines specifically designed for back problems, which should be done before and after the exercise routine.

One final word of advice: to most people, exercise means action—energy! Perspiration running down their bodies through twists, bends, jumps, sit-ups. This does not necessarily produce a fit body. Any type of exercise that leaves you feeling exhausted is not worth the complications it may create in later years, if not sooner. Any type of exercise that leaves you feeling ravenously hungry is not doing its job. After exercise you should be thirsty. In fact you should always drink some water before and after exercising. If your workout is a long one drink some water in between as well.

In conclusion, when you have a bad back the world is not going to come to an end. You *can* get it back into shape—but it won't happen overnight! Remember that it didn't get out of shape overnight. The exercises in this section will help to get you back in shape. From then on the rest is up to you.

# PROPER BREATHING FOR A BETTER BACK

Unless you are a trained singer or have studied proper breathing techniques, you don't breathe properly. The only time that most people do is when they are infants. If you look at a baby breathe you will notice almost no movement in his chest, but his little abdomen will show a continuous and gentle pumping action. He is breathing naturally. What changes that? Habits we develop throughout our growing years—bad habits of exercise and posture, and emotional stress, which is closely related to proper breathing and the nervous system.

What is needed to develop proper breathing again, the natural way, is just a little detour of our point of focus from the upper chest to the region below our rib cage where the diaphragm muscle, the most important muscle of respiration, is located. Once we understand what its location and function is, the rest is just a matter of practice until it becomes a new habit.

As illustrated, the diaphragm is a fibrous muscle sheath that separates the thorax from the abdominal area of the trunk. It is shaped like a dome in which its circular base is attached to the walls of the chest and covers the entire body from front to back. When this muscle contracts its central portion, the top of the dome moves down and inward, creating a vacuum that fills the enlarged thoracic area of the lungs with air. The voluntary contraction of the diaphragm muscle is simultaneous with the forward extension of the abdominal muscles. When the abdominal muscles are then contracted they exert a force on the vital organs they protect, an action which helps to push the diaphragm muscle back up to its dome position. This chain produces the exhaling of breathing.

At this point you may ask, why isn't chest breathing good enough? It is not a question of it being good enough, but of whether there is another way that is better. Chest breathing fills the upper part of the lungs and neglects the lower lobes, where most of our exchange of gas for blood distribution takes place. This impairs the exchange and makes the lungs work harder to provide proper oxygenation. Through diaphragmatic breathing the air is pulled all the way down to the lower lobes, the exchange takes place faster and more efficiently and the entire cardiovascular system is properly irrigated. Although the amount of oxygen consumed by the body is the same in chest breathing as it is in diaphragmatic breathing, the amount of work required by the heart and lungs is much less, allowing them to work more efficiently during exercise and contributing more to the exchanges that take part in our nervous and muscular systems.

While the exact function of the diaphragm is still not completely understood, it is known that chest breathing keeps the body's arousal mechanism on alert by causing pressure on the right vagus nerve, which

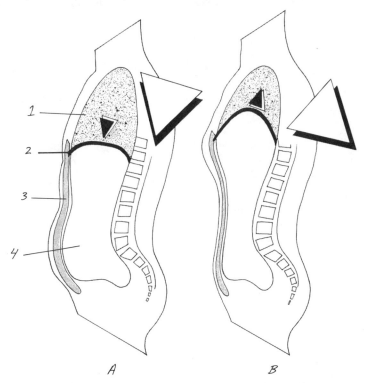

*A*                    *B*

*Figures A and B show the position of the lungs (#1) and the diaphragm muscle (#2) while breathing in and out. Notice the expansion of the abdominal muscles (#3) and abdominal cavity (#4) during inhalation (figure A), in contrast with that of exhalation (figure B).*

connects to about eighty percent of our vital organs. Phil Nuernberger writes in *Freedom from Stress: A Holistic Approach*, "As long as we breathe with the chest muscles instead of the diaphragm, we are continually creating an unnecessary level of stress."

It is important to note that proper breathing is not possible without proper postural alignment of the head, spine and pelvis. As we've seen bad postural habits are directly correlated to back problems. In cases of a habitual round back, shrunken chest or both, the ribs are cramped in front and the freedom of movement is obstructed, resulting in shallow breathing. People who habitually stick their chin forward create tightness in the chest and neck muscles, inhibiting respiration. And those with extreme swayback do not allow the abdominal muscle to perform its role in expiration, which is that of helping the rib cage to close downward and inward.

## A BREATHING EXERCISE

Do this exercise as often as you can. After a while you will get a feel for it and will be able to do it with ease.

1. Sit up straight. Keep your upper chest high, but not jutting out as in a military stance. Try to get a feeling of support from the trunk muscles, which will make you feel as if you are sitting taller. You probably are. Close your eyes.

2. Lace your fingers together and place the palms of your hands directly under the rib cage, where the diaphragm is located. Keep the stomach in but not forcibly tight. If you are really sitting tall they will probably have the right amount of contraction.

3. Open your mouth wide and close it, trying to relax the lower jaw. Do this a couple of times, then keep your mouth open.

4. Visualize a dome inside your chest. Hold on to that image throughout this exercise and don't allow any other thought to enter your mind.

5. Close your mouth and as you inhale through your nose, picture the top of the dome going down into your hands. Feel the pressure against the palms of your hands while at the same time you feel the air travel into your lower back (remember that the diaphragm extends from front to back).

6. Press in lightly and visualize the dome going back to its original position as the air flows out of your mouth.

7. Repeat as many times as you want. You will feel the difference almost immediately.

## PROPER BREATHING WHILE DOING BACK EXERCISES

If you follow the above instructions you will soon be able to use your diaphragm properly without having to place your hands below your ribs. If used during the Tension Release Exercises and the Daily Rehab Conditioners, diaphragmatic breathing will intensify their positive effects.

1. Practice the breathing exercise outlined above a few times before exercising. As you do so try to clear your mind of all thoughts other than that of getting your back in shape.

2. Keep your jaw relaxed, with mouth slightly open at all times.

3. Inhale through the nose.

4. Exhale through the mouth, and try to take at least twice as long to exhale as you did to inhale.

# IMAGINED ACTION

When I was a child my parents, who are both in the medical profession, thought it would be a good idea for me to take dance lessons as rehabilitation for an asthmatic and a previous poliomyelitic condition. Each morning our teacher managed to scare her reluctant pupils into practicing classical feet positions at the ballet barre. Her favorite phrase, which captured the essence of her teaching was "Think! Let your brain do the dancing first; then just point your feet and go." Concentrating on dance at age twelve was definitely harder for me than pointing my feet, although that, too, was not done without difficulty—as time would tell, my feet were never made for ballet dancing. And although that was something my teacher failed to notice, she *was* right about one thing—when it comes to movement, it pays to think before doing.

Movement is a neuro-muscular action even when it hasn't been preceded by conscious thought. But when you think before doing, the result is usually a smoother action that requires less output of unnecessary energy and results in better and more efficient cooperation of the areas surrounding the movement's point of origin. This in itself reduces the chance of malfunction or injury to the muscles that are executing the action. In both my dance and fitness classes I have seen the benefits of concentrating while exercising and visualizing a movement before it is executed. Although this theory is more useful to dancers and others who have an above average knowledge of the mechanics of their skeletal and muscular system, I have also seen the improvement in nondancers who had previously only thought of exercise as a means of sweating and getting their bodies "worked out." This attitude of exercising without thinking about what you're doing is, unfortunately, more prevalent now because of the increased popularity of aerobic dancing classes. In many of these classes enthusiastic dance students, who oftentimes become overnight teachers, will put a group of people eager to shed some pounds and improve their cardiovascular system through a series of body motions which are more akin to clever jogging steps. Too often these teachers have more choreographic talent than anatomical knowledge and are unable to advise their students on what they should and shouldn't do, according to each student's degree of fitness. The consequences of this aerobic dance euphoria

is seen in the offices of orthopedic doctors, osteopaths and chiropra..
Although dancing to improve cardiovascular endurance is certainly more
invigorating and enjoyable than a brisk walk, the latter is just as good and,
depending on the teacher, certainly much safer for the average person who
hasn't exercised regularly and whose muscles lack proper tone. Referred
back pain (that which is hard to localize) from aerobic dancing follows the
same vicious cycle that plagues many weekend athletes! Pain hits, the
person stops activity until pain subsides and then starts up again where he
left off until the pain hits again.

The use of "imagined action" is used in several forms and variations
throughout the country by physiatrists (doctors of physical medicine),
exercise physiologists and physical therapists with patients undergoing
rehabilitation. It is, to my knowledge, seldom used in dance or exercise
studios. One reason is because it is best done on a one-to-one basis and
with people who are going through physical rehabilitation after injury or
surgery. It is hard to do in large groups not only because it's time consuming, but because the instructor must constantly create a series of images
that each student can respond to—not everyone responds the same way to
each image. I hope in this section you'll learn enough about the application of imagined action to do it yourself.

The role of the power of the mind over body has been an area of
tremendous research and speculation throughout the last few years. How
much or how little our mind can influence physical actions is yet to be
determined. Dr. Carl Simonton wrote in *Getting Well Again* (J. P. Tarcher)
that today imagined action is even being employed by doctors in the
treatment of cancer patients—and with some success. My first introduction to imagined action was through articles written by Mabel Elsworth
Todd and Dr. Lulu Sweigard. I then saw their principles of body mechanics
put into practice by professional ballroom dance teams which I frequently
coach. While in all forms of dance proper posture and maintaining equilibrium are essential, in ballroom dance it is especially important, for the
equilibrium of two people must be maintained evenly throughout movement and their lines of gravity and centers of gravity must merge as one.

Throughout the following chapters you also will become aware of the
tremendous value of imagined action in exercise, alleviation of pain
and development of better postural habits and body mechanics. I have
seen the effects of its application in people whose chests were caved in,
whose backs were hunched or whose coordination was almost nonexis-
tent. There are as many images that can improve our bodies and its
functions as there are minds that can create them. For the purpose of this
book I will provide you with some suggested images to help you carry out
the exercises and receive the best results possible.

## APPLYING IMAGINED ACTION TO
## EXERCISES INVOLVING THE LEGS

*Fishing Pole:* (Thigh flexion over body/straight leg lift)

Whenever any of the exercises call for you to lie on your back with your leg raised, think of your entire leg (thigh, leg, and foot) as a fishing pole. The foot is the fish, while the leg is the line. The thigh is the pole which ends as a handle (the hip joint, from which all motions originate). Imagined action takes place by your visualizing that in order to bring the foot closer to the body, it is your action at the handle, or hip joint, which raises the pole and "reels" it in.

In movements where you are called to lift one leg straight up from the floor, think of the entire leg as the fishing pole that rises from the hip joint.

FOR THE ABDOMINAL MUSCLES

*The Aluminum Foil:* (Lower and upper body curls)

For any of the exercises that concentrate on the lower and upper abdominal muscles, think of your abdomen as a crumpled piece of aluminum foil which you are about to smooth out: You open up the paper (as when you lie on the floor) and place your fingers on the center of the paper (your abdomen) and start soothing from the center outward (from the stomach to the legs or from the stomach to the head).

ALL-PURPOSE IMAGE

Any image that helps you to realize that all the movements for these exercises originate in the abdominal area will contribute to better execution. For instance, whenever the legs move their movement starts at the hip joint. If the torso moves forward, back, or to the side while you are lying on the floor, it does so from the area surrounding the navel. If the torso bends forward from a standing position it does so from the hip joint, *not* from the waist. If the arms move up, down, or extend in any direction they do so from their attachment point, the shoulders and shoulder blades.

As one last reminder I will add that proper use of images is not possible without good breathing and relaxation. The following tips on relaxation are taken from Dr. Herbert Benson's *The Relaxation Response* (William Morrow), an excellent book in which he explains how relaxation can be achieved through meditation.

—In quiet surroundings sit in a comfortable position with eyes closed.

—Relax all muscles, starting at the feet and working up to the face.

—Breathe through the nose and on exhaling say the word "one" slowly and silently.

—Do not compete with yourself. Maintain a passive attitude in trying to become relaxed. The harder you try the less chance you'll have of becoming truly relaxed.

—Practice relaxation as often as you can.

# THE TENSION-RELEASE EXERCISES

The Tension-Release Exercises (TRE) have a dual purpose: mind-muscle preparation and cool-down. The purpose of these exercises is to get your mind, your respiratory, circulatory and muscular systems ready to coordinate their forces for the execution of the daily set of back exercises, called the Daily Rehab Conditioners (DRC), which are found later in this section. After you complete the Daily Rehab Conditioners, you should once again do the Tension Release Exercises. This repetition is necessary to help stretch muscles, tendons and ligaments a little further, and will also help to release the tensions that often build up during exercise. In short, they will act as a cool-down, even though the DRC are not overtaxing—they are primarily stretches for your back and hip muscles to help increase their flexibility and elasticity, and improve muscle tone.

I will again remind you to read the instructions a couple of times for each exercise while looking at the photos before doing them.

*Note: The Tension Release Exercises must be coordinated with proper breathing. In performing these exercises one must remember to inhale through the nose and exhale through the mouth.*

### *TRE #1. Torso Lift*

*Purpose*: To roll up the torso while in the sitting position until it is straight, with the head relaxed down on the chest.

*Step One*: Begin in a sitting position with the torso bent over the thighs and the arms hanging loosely at your sides. Inhale deeply through the nose. Hold it. As you exhale through the mouth start rolling up and stop when you feel the lower back come closer to the back of the chair.

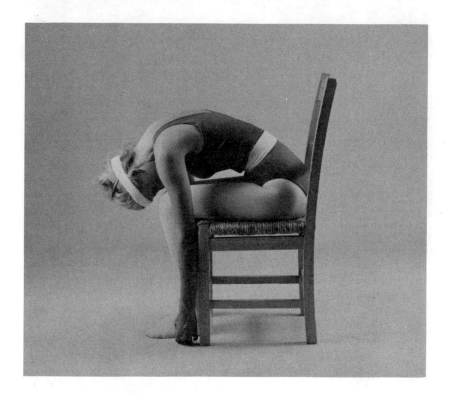

*Step Two*: Inhale deeply. Hold it. As you exhale continue rolling up until you feel the middle back get closer to the back of the chair. Keep shoulders, head and arms relaxed.

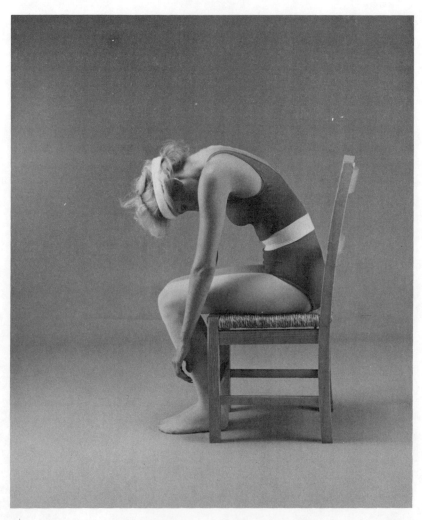

*Imagined Action*: Picture the spine's skeletal structure and as you roll up visualize placing each vertebra on top of the other, one at a time.

*Step Three*: Inhale deeply. Hold it. As you exhale continue rolling up until you finally feel the spine straight, the shoulder blades in place. Keep your head down and let the arms hang loosely at your sides.

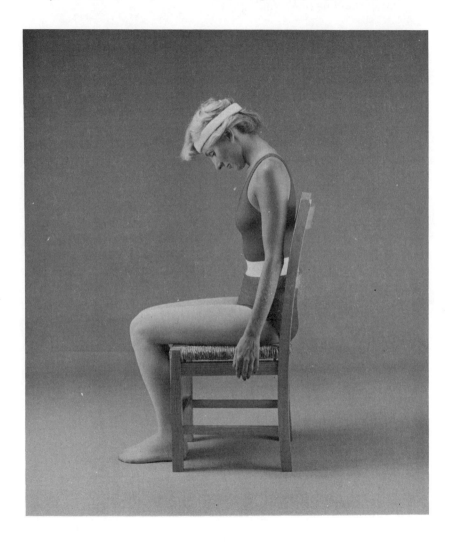

*TRE #2. Neck Roll*

*Purpose*: To relax all the muscles of the head, face and neck, this can be done standing or sitting.

*Step One*: Beginning with the head held up, inhale. Hold it. Exhale slowly as you roll the neck clockwise until the chin is over the right shoulder. Keep arms at your side, chest high, stomach relaxed and the spine straight. Only the neck should move.

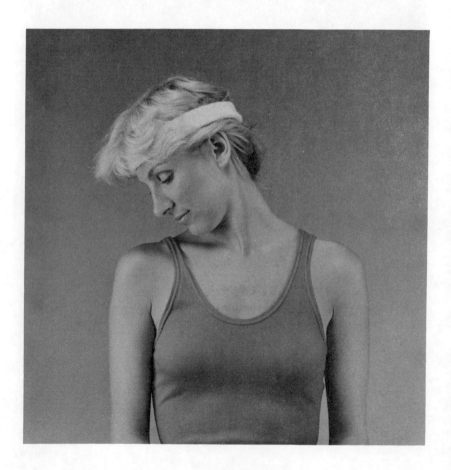

*Step Two*: Exhale as the head rolls back until you are looking at the ceiling. Stop in that position and inhale.

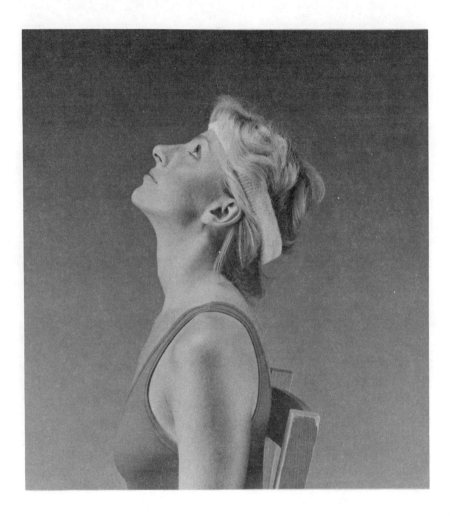

*Step Three*: Exhale as you roll the head over to the left shoulder. Stop when the chin is over it and inhale.

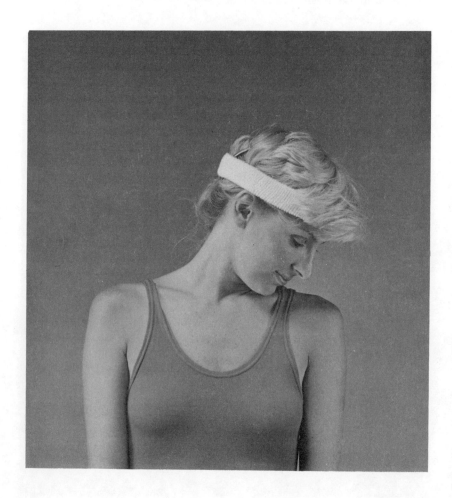

*Step Four*: Exhale as you bring the head down and the chin is touching the upper chest. Inhale, then start the entire procedure counterclockwise.

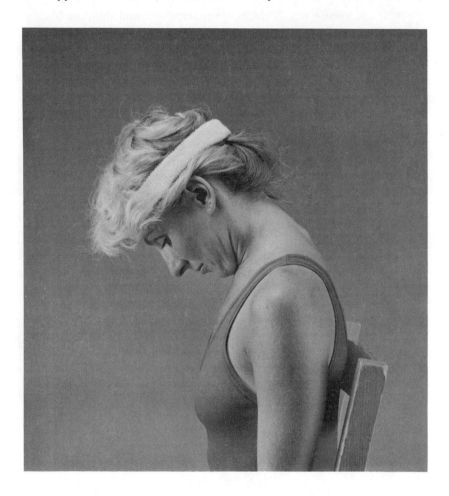

### TRE #3. Shoulder Shrug

*Purpose*: To release tension from upper shoulders and shoulder blades.

*Execution*: Right after completing the head roll and while the head is down take a deep breath and as you exhale bring the shoulders as close to your ears as possible. Then bring them down and lift the head, being sure the back of the head is aligned over the spine.

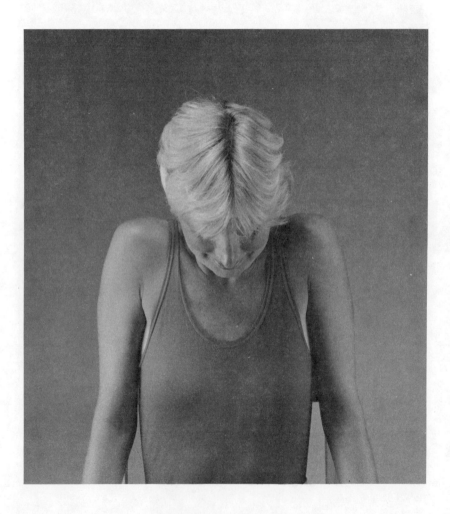

## TRE #4. Combination Stretch

*Purpose*: To work all the major muscle groups of the back, the stomach, the shoulders and the thighs.

*Preparation*: Stand straight with fingers laced on the stomach. Inhale deeply and feel the air press the stomach against the hands.

*Step One*: Exhale as you bend the knees. Turn the palms of the hands over and extend the arms downward while pulling the stomach in, rounding the upper back and moving the head down into the loop formed by the arms. This time the hips are going back as if you were going to sit on the chair. You should feel a gentle stretch on the back as the arms extend forward.

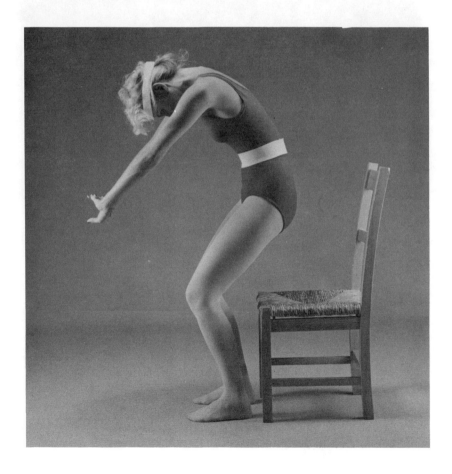

*Step Two*: Inhale as you return to the starting position, once again feeling the air press against your hands. Keep your body and spine straight.

*Step Three*: Exhale as you again bend the knees but this time turn the palms of your hands to the ceiling. Keep the head down.

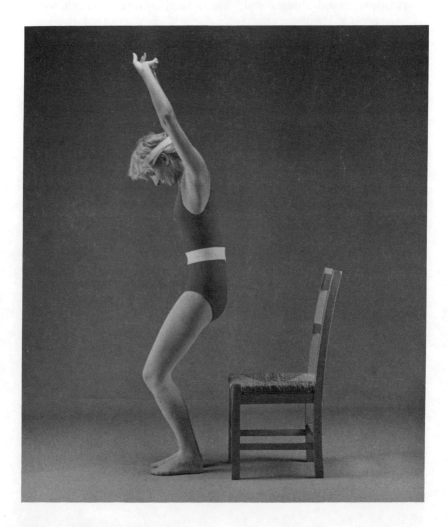

*Step Four*: Inhale as you return to the starting position.

*Imagined Action*: The idea here is to visualize a rubber band being pulled at both ends and feeling its center section thin out as it stretches.

## TRE #5. Total Back Stretch

*Purpose*: To strengthen the psoas major and hamstring muscles and to release tension from the hip and groin areas.

*Preparation*: Face the chair, placing both hands on the seat. Feet should be parallel, no wider apart than the width of the hips. Start with the knees slightly bent and the back as flat as possible. Take a deep breath and let the stomach hang loose.

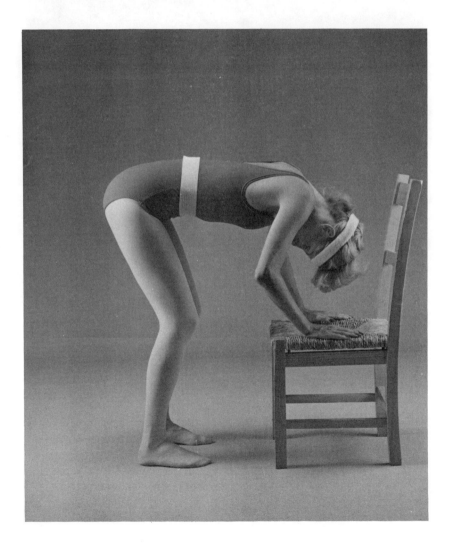

*Step One*: As you exhale bend the knees and the elbows while placing your head on the seat of the chair.

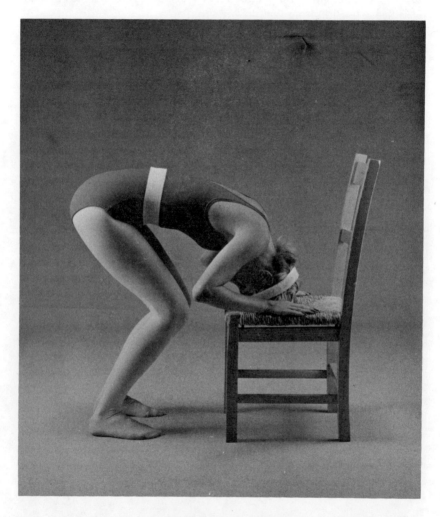

*Step Two*: Inhale deeply. Hold it and exhale while remaining in that position. The closer your chest is to your thighs the more you'll feel the stretch, but don't force your chest downward—let the movement of your breathing bring the chest closer to the thighs. You will see and feel the difference after about a week of doing this exercise.

*Step Three*: Inhale again. Hold it.

*Step Four*: As you exhale press down on the seat of the chair with your arms and slowly push your torso up until your arms and your legs are straight.

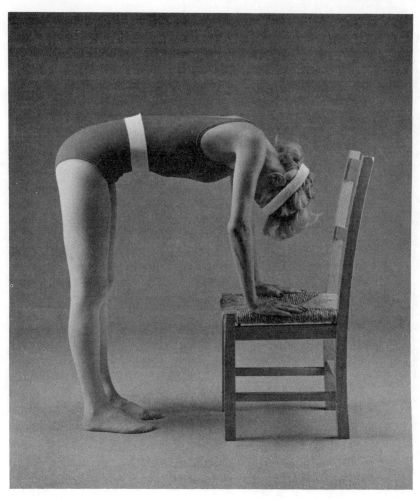

*Step Five*: Inhale. Hold it. Now exhale fast and hard (as if you were trying to blow air into the chair's seat). Feel the stomach pull in and the back round.

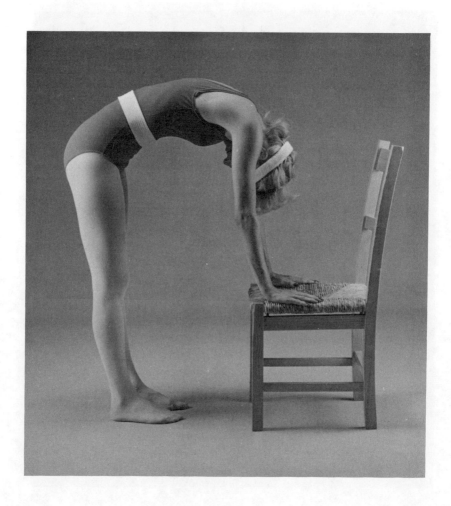

*Step Six*: Straighten up as you complete exhaling, one vertebra at a time.

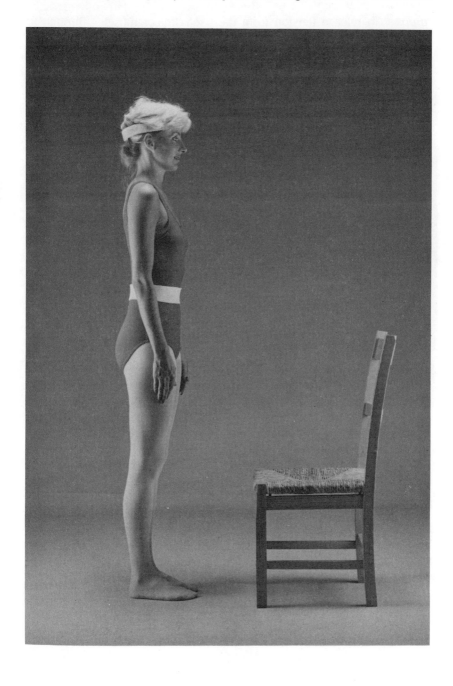

## *TRE #6. Iliopsoas Stretch*

*Purpose*: To release tension from the psoas major muscles through a combination of deep breathing, applied pressure and relaxation.

*Starting Position*: Lie on your back with legs extended.

*Step One*: As you inhale bring one knee up to the chest and hold it with both hands.

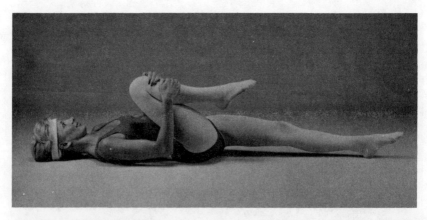

*Step Two*: Take eight slow counts to exhale. As you do so apply light but continuous, downward pressure on your leg, bringing the thigh closer to the chest. Make sure that the extended leg stays straight and does not come off the floor at the hip joint. If the hip joint starts to come up, keep the knee bent at whichever level you had reached before the other hip started to move up.

Switch legs and repeat the exercise. Now you are ready for the Daily Rehab Conditioners.

A FINAL NOTE: Although these exercises should be done before and after the DRC, it is beneficial to do them any time when stress builds up. For those who must spend a lot of time sitting these exercises will also aid circulation. If they can be done a couple of times throughout the day, you will find that they'll help your neck and back from getting too stiff.

# THE DAILY REHAB CONDITIONERS (DRC)

These exercises are designed to reduce lower back tension by progressively increasing the range of motion of the hip joint and strengthening the abdominal and back muscles. All of the exercises are divided into four groups which alternately work the groin, hip and buttocks area; the lower abdomen and the lower back; and the chest, middle and upper back.

### Who Can Benefit from the Daily Rehab Conditioners?

The DRC are easy to learn and do; they can be done by anyone whose back pain has been diagnosed as due to a mechanical muscular condition. If back pain is due to a mechanical *skeletal* condition, such as a worn facet joint or a combination of conditions, such as a worn facet joint that has inflamed a disc, the DRC would still be beneficial, but you should check with your doctor before doing them. Remember that simply being told that "You need to exercise" is not enough. If you have this book on hand show it to your doctor and ask him or her if your type of back pain could benefit from these exercises. Most likely the answer will be yes. If your back pain is due to a pinched nerve, regardless of the reason, also check with your doctor. If your doctor gives you the go-ahead and you are not feeling pain, *follow the progression but just do one set of each exercise throughout.* Do not do the suggested number of repetitions if you have a pinched nerve.

OVERWEIGHT

Needless to say, if your back has started to scream pain because you have neglected it and you are overweight, the first thing you must try to do is lose weight. One advantage to being heavier is that when you exercise you burn more calories faster than a skinny person in the same amount of time and with the same type of exercise. Nevertheless, exercise alone will not burn enough calories to make a permanent difference unless it is backed by proper nutrition. The DRC can be done by overweight people but might prove difficult for obese people once they reach the third week. My advice is to continue to try all of the exercises. If one particular exercise seems too

**91**

difficult, don't attempt to do the suggested number of repetitions, but do at least one.

For people with either of these conditions the DRC can bring tremendous benefits. But the degree of improvement possible varies as much as does the age of the people who are afflicted by them. Have your doctor review these exercises before you begin. If they're approved, follow the progression as indicated for the first four weeks, then continue to do them at least three times a week.

## How to Make the DRC Work

The exercises are most beneficial when done in the morning and in the evening. If, however, you are one of the millions who must get up and run to work each morning, I suggest you do the Tension Release Exercises (TRE) only (total time: five to ten minutes). Then do the TRE and the DRC group in the evening before dinner.

One thing you should *not* do is to exercise some mornings or afternoons while skipping others. You are better off not exercising at all. These exercises are designed to be done with continuity; doing them on and off could actually hurt you.

The exercises are divided into groups of four which are repeated for seven days before a new group of four is added to the routine. The results of this gradual conditioning will allow your body, by the fourth week, to do sixteen exercises in total. The completed workout should take between twenty-five to thirty minutes. About five minutes are added each week—something to remember if you must set an alarm clock every morning.

## The Overload Progression Principle

Only by adding exercises on a weekly basis and increasing repetitions on a daily basis will you reap the benefits of the Overload Principle, discussed on page 44. Then, once your body learns the mechanics of each exercise, it can practically do them while you're asleep.

Make sure you follow the instructions and stick to the progression even if you were the town's All-American before your first attack of back pain.

Each exercise is broken down into a series of steps which, together, form a set. Besides adding four new exercises every week, you also will be increasing the number of sets of each exercise done each day. For example, if today is the first day in which you are going to exercise you will do each exercise given for the first week one time—this is one set. Tomorrow, your second day, you will do each exercise in the first week two times—this will constitute two sets. At the end of the first week you will have worked up to seven sets of each exercise, which you should continue to do seven times for the following three weeks. You will also be adding four new exercises on the first day of each week.

Let's say you are on the third day of your second week. Besides continuing to do seven repetitions of the first four exercises, you should also be doing three repetitions of the second set of four which you learned three days ago—the start of the second week.

Remember to do the six Tension Release Exercises in Section Two before you begin the DRC.

## THE DAILY REHAB CONDITIONERS
## WEEK ONE

*The First Day*: It is normal to feel apprehensive about anything that is tried for the first time. If you have just gotten over a bout of back pain your apprehensions regarding exercise are well justified. Be aware that there is a marked difference between pain and discomfort. You may feel some discomfort during the first couple of days, or as you increase repetitions. Discomfort doesn't last very long as your body relaxes into the exercises— but if real pain is felt at any time, stop. Remember to do these exercises slowly, especially during the first couple of days.

THE TOTAL REST POSITION (TRP)
This is the basic position from which we will begin many of the

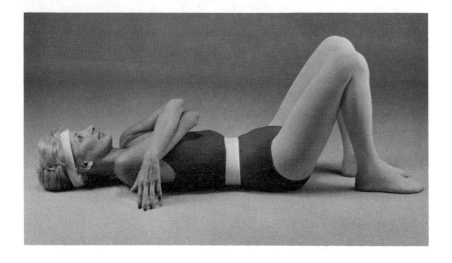

exercises. Lie on the floor with the arms wrapped over the chest, fingers touching the floor. This induces release of tight muscles in the upper back and shoulder blades. Some people will not be able to hold this position for long before they feel their elbows start to slide outward. This is a sign of tight back and chest muscles. Those with overdeveloped muscular frames will also find this hard to sustain.

The knees are bent, preferably at a 90 degree angle; the feet should be kept as close to the pelvis as possible in a parallel position and in direct line under the knees. The knees should be in a direct forward line from the hip joint. Maintaining this position will also be difficult for those with tight hip muscles.

While in this position concentrate on breathing deeply, taking twice as long for exhalation. Imagine that the spine is expanding in a straight line from the pelvis.

### Exercise #1: Two-Way Slide

*Starting Position*: TRP.

*Step One*: Take a deep breath. As you exhale slide the heel of one leg forward until the leg is straight. Keep the ankle flexed (foot pointing to the ceiling) until the leg is fully extended.

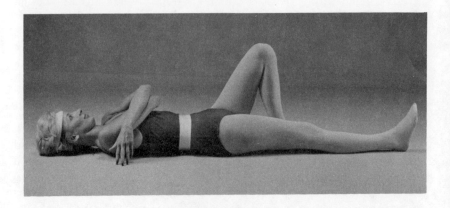

*Step Two*: Inhale again and slowly extend the foot until the toe is pointed.

*Step Three*: As you exhale slide the foot back up toward the pelvis, bringing the thigh over the chest. As you do this you will feel your lower back get closer to the floor. Do not let the buttocks muscle on the side you are working lift off the floor.

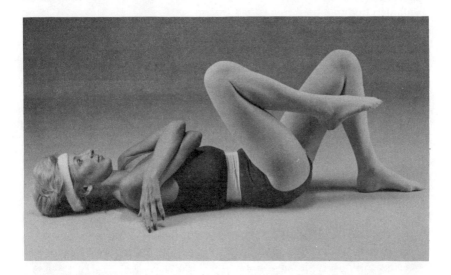

*Step Four*: Inhale as you place the foot on the floor and resume the starting position.

Repeat on the other side.

### Exercise #2: Lower Body Curl

*Starting Position*: TRP

It is also known as a Pelvic Tuck, Tilt or an Abdominal Contraction. I, and many others, call it a curl because its execution should be visualized as if the tail bone or coccyx curls into the stomach—like the tail of a scorpion. This movement is important because it causes the contraction of the abdominal muscles. You will see the further benefits of this exercise when you start doing other exercises that target the abdominal area.

*Step One*: Take a deep breath. As you exhale pull in the stomach, forcing the lower back to press against the floor; the buttocks will come off the floor. Hold that position for six counts. Keep tightening the stomach as you exhale.

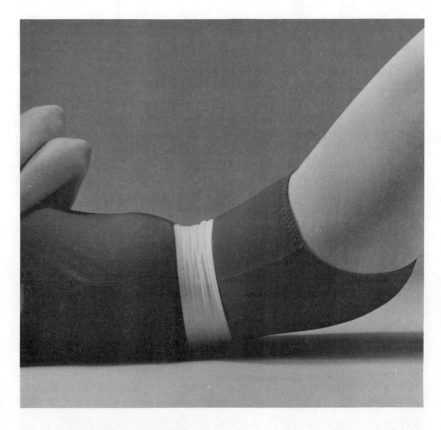

*Step Two*: Inhale as you release the tightness and place the buttocks back on the floor. Do this to a count of eight.

*Note*: This simple exercise is the key to the successful execution of the exercises that follow in this group. It is very effective as a postural exercise and as a preliminary step to the strenghtening of the stomach muscles and those of the lower back.

## Exercise #3: Lumbar Flex

*Starting Position*: Fetal Cuddle. Lie on your side with both knees bent, one leg resting on top of the other.

*Step One*: Inhale. As you exhale bring the upper knee up as if to touch the upper shoulder.

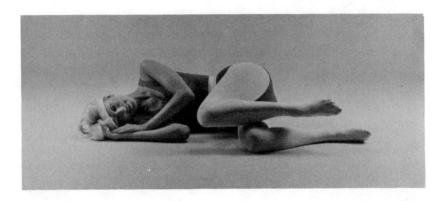

*Step Two*: Inhale. Slide the upper leg down until it is fully extended with toe pointed.

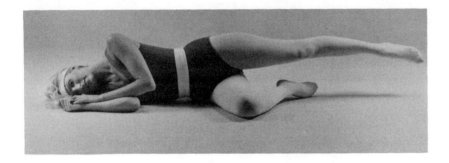

### *Exercise #4: Buttocks Pinch*

*Starting Position*: Lie face down on the floor with your forehead resting on
   your hands.

*Step One*: Inhale. As you exhale let the heels of both feet roll outward as
   you pinch or contract the buttocks muscles. Hold the contraction for
   seven counts and release it on the eighth.
   Now turn on your back and do the TRE in reverse order.

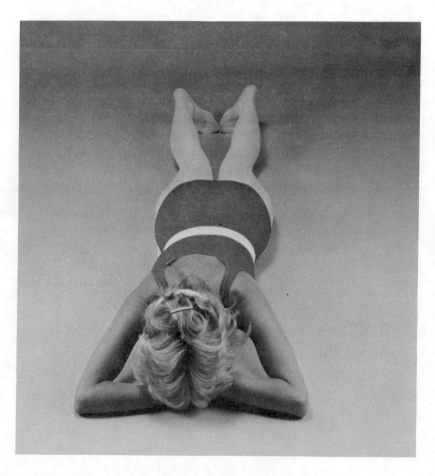

This completes the exercises for the first day. Remember that each day
you will add one repetition of each exercise until the seventh day, then you
will add this set to the second week of your routine.

## WEEK TWO

**#1.** Do seven repetitions of the Two-Way Slide

**#2. *New Exercise: Thigh Flexion***

*Starting Position*: TRP with arms alongside the body.

*Step One*: Inhale. As you exhale lift the thigh of one leg over the stomach. The foot is relaxed—neither flexed nor pointed.

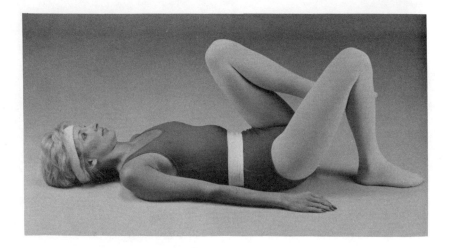

*Step Two*: Inhale as you place the foot back down in the starting position.

Repeat with the other leg.

*Step Three*: Take another breath. As you exhale tighten the stomach muscles and lift both thighs over the chest. Try to keep the legs parallel and avoid rotation by keeping them in a straight angle with the hip joint.

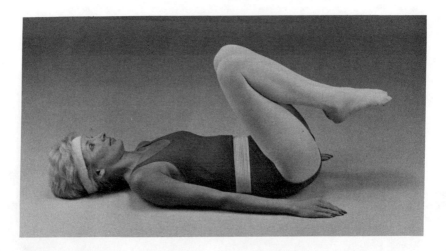

*Step Four*: Inhale as you place them back down.
Repeat the last two steps.

**#3.** Do seven repetitions of the Lower Body Curl

## #4. New Exercise: Upper Body Curl

*Starting Position*: TRP.

*Step One*: Inhale. As you exhale lift the chin to the chest and contract the abdominal muscles. As the stomach tightens continue to curl up by lifting the shoulder blades off the floor. Try to hold for twenty counts.

Although the Upper Body Curl lifts the head, shoulders and shoulder blades off the floor, the movement is produced by a contraction of the mid-abdominal muscles. The benefits of one slow curl done as previously described is said to equal the effect of five sit-ups.

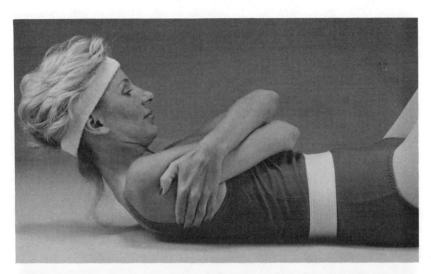

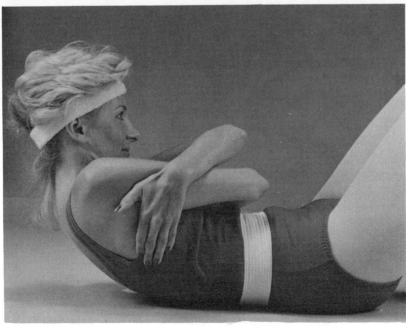

*Step Two*: Inhale as you roll back down.

*Note*: Leave the chin forward as you add repetitions to this exercise. Too often the forward and backward movement of the head is used as momentum for the curl. This not only takes away from the strengthening purpose of the movement but can provoke cervical tension and pain.

**#5.** Do seven repetitions of the Lumbar Flex.

**#6. *New Exercise: Front Extension***

*Starting Position*: Fetal Cuddle (see Lumbar Flex).

*Step One*: Inhale as you bring the upper knee up as if to touch the upper shoulder.

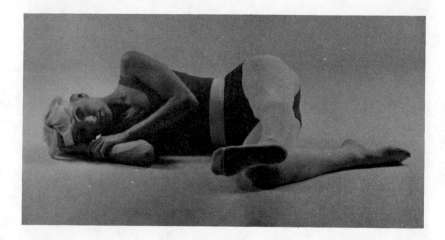

*Step Two*: Exhale as you extend the leg forward as close to hip level as possible. Keep the foot flexed.

*Step Three*: Inhale. Return the leg to a resting position.

**#7.** Do seven repetitions of the Buttocks Pinch.

### #8. New Exercise: The Round Back

*Starting Position*: Kneel on your hands and knees with weight distributed evenly between the two. This is called the Four Prone Position.

*Step One*: Start with the back as flat as possible (as if you were a table). Take a deep breath and as you exhale round the back and contract the abdominal muscles. Keep the chin as close to the chest as possible.

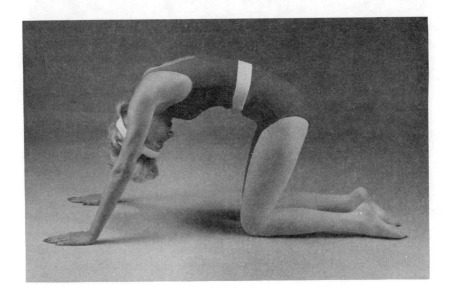

*Step Two*: Inhale as you bring the chin up and move the hips back over the feet, as if you were trying to sit on your calves. Even though the lower back will try to arch keep it as flat as possible.

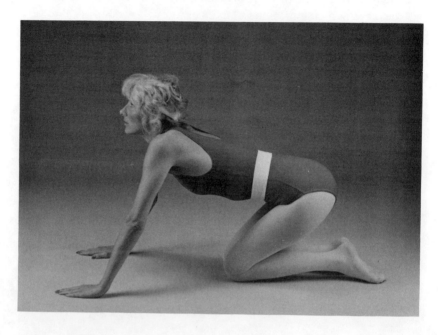

Cool off gradually by doing the Tension Release Exercises in reverse order.

## WEEK THREE

**#1.** Do seven repetitions of the Two-Way Slide.

**#2.** Do seven repetitions of the Thigh Flex.

**#3. *New Exercise: Leg Lift***

*Starting Position*: TRP.

*Step One*: Inhale. As you exhale slide the heel of one leg down until the leg is straight. Keep the foot flexed.

*Step Two*: Inhale as you raise the leg. Do not lift it any higher than you can without keeping your leg straight. For our purposes the most beneficial way of executing this movement is by thinking of narrowing the angle between the thigh bone and the hip joint as the leg goes up, instead of thinking of simply raising the foot.

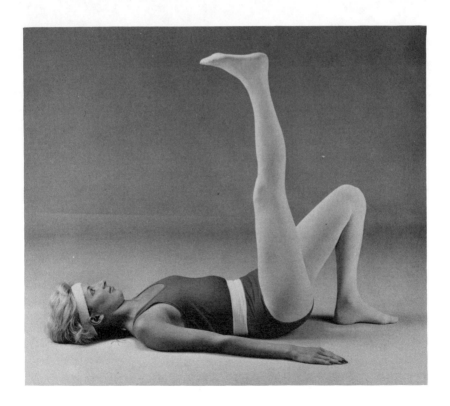

*Step Three*: As you exhale concentrate on narrowing that angle even more. Bend the knee, bringing the thigh directly over the chest. Return the foot to the starting position. Repeat on the other side.

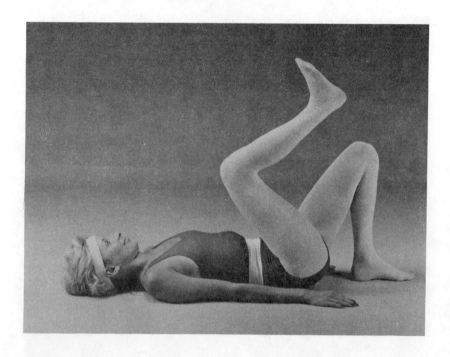

**#4.** Do seven repetitions of the Lower Body Curl.

**#5.** Do seven repetitions of the Upper Body Curl.

### #6. New Exercise: Lower Body Lift

*Starting Position:* TRP with arms alongside the body.

*Step One:* Start as if you were going to do another Lower Body Curl, but continue lifting the torso until you form a straight line from your knees to the middle of the back. Inhale throughout the upward movement.

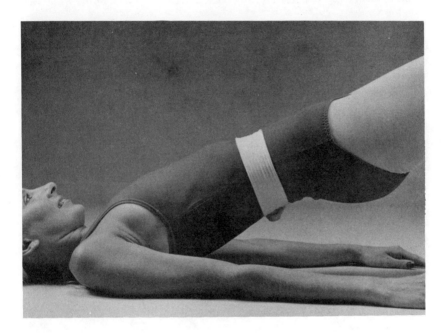

*Step Two:* Exhale as you lower the back onto the floor, starting from the top of the back down to the buttocks. Do this slowly, as if you were placing one vertabra at a time on the floor.

**#7.** Do seven repetitions of the Lumbar Flex.

**#8.** Do seven repetitions of the Front Extension on one side. Don't turn over to do it on the other side until you also do the new exercise (Thigh Rotation) on that side.

### #9. New Exercise: Thigh Rotation

*Starting Position*: Lie on your side with both legs straight. The upper leg should be extended forward at about hip level. It is important that the body is well anchored so that nothing moves except the entire leg. Place the hand of the upper arm firmly on the floor in front of your stomach. Let your body lean forward so that the arm acts as a brace. This will keep you from rolling back and twisting your spine while the leg works.

*Step One*: Lift the leg off the floor and turn it so that the toes point towards the floor (inward rotation). Hold for 10 counts. Now turn the heel toward the floor so that the toes point upward (outward rotation). Hold for 10 counts. Repeat on the other side.

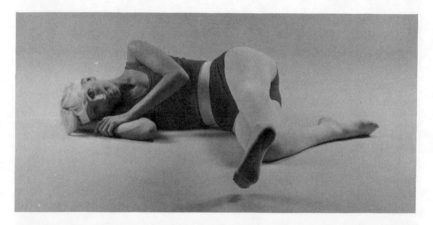

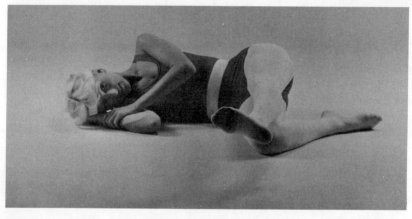

**#10.** Do seven repetitions of the Buttocks Pinch.

**#11.** Do seven repetitions of the Round Back.

**#12. *New Exercise: Back-Chest Stretch***

*Starting Position*: Four Prone Position (see The Round Back)

*Step One*: Inhale. As you exhale try to sit back on your calves. Let your chest rest on your thighs and allow the arms to be as fully extended as possible. The arms shouldn't be any farther apart than shoulder-width.

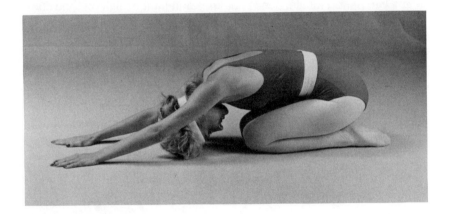

*Step Two*: Inhale as you return to the starting position. Now do the Tension Release Exercises in reverse order for a cool-down.

## WEEK FOUR

**#1.** Do seven repetitions of the Two-Way Slide.

**#2.** Do seven repetitions of the Thigh Flexion.

**#3.** Do seven repetitions of the Leg Lift.

**#4. *New Exercise: High Extension***

*Starting Position*: TRP with arms alongside the body. This exercise is the
exact reverse of the Leg Lift.

*Step One*: As you inhale, bend your knee and lift the thigh over the chest.
Flex your foot.

*Step Two*: Exhale and extend the leg. Point the foot as the leg reaches full
extension. Keep the abdominal muscles pressing against the lower
back; don't allow the buttocks to be lifted off the floor by the extended
leg.

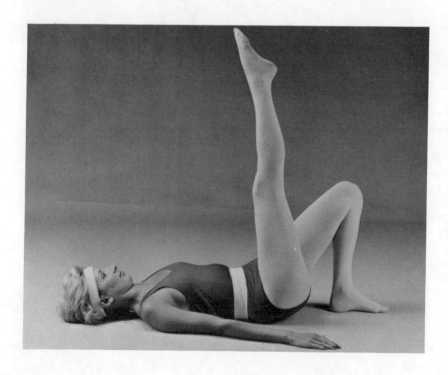

*Step Three*: Inhale as you bend the knee; exhale as leg is returned to the starting position. Repeat on the other side.

**#5.** Do seven repetitions of the Lower Body Curl.

**#6.** Do seven repetitions of the Upper Body Curl.

**#7.** Do seven repetitions of the Lower Body Lift.

**#8. *New Exercise: Two-Way Curl***

*Starting Position*: TRP with hands laced behind neck.

*Step One*: Inhale as you bring both knees toward the chest. Buttocks should not be completely lifted off the floor.

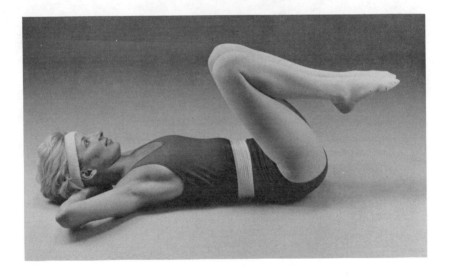

*Step Two*: Exhale as you curl up, closing elbows to touch the knees. (If you can't touch elbow to knee don't worry. It's the direction and the effort that's important—not the contact.)

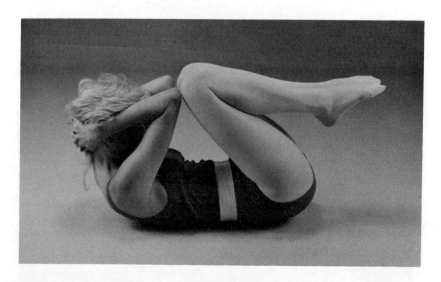

*Step Three*: Inhale as you bring both feet down to the starting position.

*Step Four*: Exhale as you roll the back down slowly.

*#9.* Do seven repetitions of the Lumbar Flex.

*#10.* Do seven repetitions of the Front Extension.

*#11.* Do seven repetitions of the Thigh Rotation.

### #12. New Exercise: Final Cuddle

*Starting Position*: TRC with arms at your sides.

*Step One*: Bring both knees to your chest and wrap your arms around them. Inhale, and as you exhale apply light pressure with your hands against the legs, trying to bring them closer to the chest. The head stays on the floor.

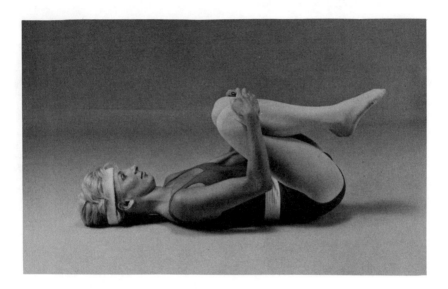

**#13.** Do seven repetitions of the Buttocks Pinch.

**#14.** Do seven repetitions of the Round Back.

**#15.** Do seven repetitions of the Back-Chest Stretch.

### #16. New Exercise: The Half Cobra

*Starting Position*: Lie on the floor, face down, with hands next to your shoulders.

*Step One*: Inhale. As you exhale lift your upper torso. Use your arms for balance but try not to press against the floor. The idea is to let the muscles of your back get you to this position. Keep the chest relaxed and the shoulders down.

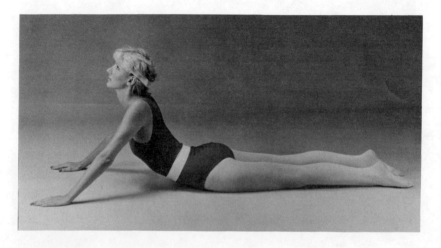

*Step Two*: Inhale as you roll down inch by inch.
Cool off by doing the Tension Release Exercises in reverse order.

## THE DAILY REHAB CONDITIONERS
## FOUR-WEEK PROGRESSION CHART

| *Week One* | *Week Two* | *Week Three* | *Week Four* |
|---|---|---|---|
| 1) Two-Way Slide | 1) Two-Way Slide | 1) Two-Way Slide | 1) Two-Way Slide |
| | 2) Thigh Flexion | 2) Thigh Flexion | 2) Thigh Flexion |
| | | 3) Leg Lift | 3) Leg Lift |
| | | | 4) High Extension |
| 2) Lower Body Curl | 3) Lower Body Curl | 4) Lower Body Curl | 5) Lower Body Curl |
| | 4) Upper Body Curl | 5) Upper Body Curl | 6) Upper Body Curl |
| | | 6) Lower Body Lift | 7) Lower Body Lift |
| | | | 8) Two-Way Curl |
| 3) Lumbar Flex | 5) Lumbar Flex | 7) Lumbar Flex | 9) Lumbar Flex |
| | 6) Front Extension | 8) Front Extension | 10) Front Extension |
| | | 9) Thigh Rotation | 11) Thigh Rotation |
| | | | 12) Final Cuddle |
| 4) Buttocks Pinch | 7) Buttocks Pinch | 10) Buttocks Pinch | 13) Buttocks Pinch |
| | 8) Round Back | 11) Round Back | 14) Round Back |
| | | 12) Back-Chest Stretch | 15) Back-Chest Stretch |
| | | | 16) Half Cobra |

# SUPPLEMENTAL EXERCISES FOR PREVENTION OF FURTHER BACK PAIN

The following exercises should only be done by those who have followed the Daily Rehabilitation Routine, or have been advised by their physician to do exercises for better abdominal and back strength.

The key to developing muscle strength lies in regularity of exercise and the gradual increase of repetitions of an exercise. The exercises in this section are intended for adults who have not previously exercised much. If you don't find these exercises difficult enough for you, you'll find more advanced exercises in my book *20 Days To a Trimmer Torso* (Simon & Schuster).

Notice that in each of the following exercises I have recommended the number of repetitions you should build to in a four-week period. For the best possible results these exercises should be done at least twice a week; three times a week is preferable.

If you are over fifty-five years of age and not in very good shape my suggestion is that you cut the recommended number of repetitions in half to start, but try to stick to doing them three times a week. As we get older we should exercise more frequently than when we were younger, but not as intensely.

1. Start with three sets of ten repetitions of the Upper Body Curl (see page 100). Rest one minute between sets. Add five repetitions each week.

2) The Abdominal Cross

*Starting Position*: TRP.

Extend one leg upward and try to touch the big toe with the opposite hand. You should feel abdominal muscles contract as you reach across to do so. Do not lift the torso beyond the middle back. Return to the TRP and repeat with the other leg and side.

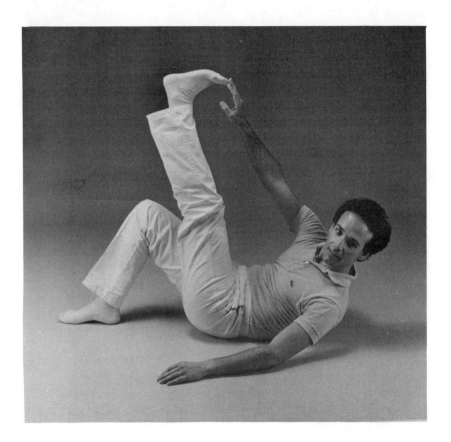

Start with three sets of ten repetitions (five foot touches on each side), resting a minute between sets. Add six more repetitions each week.

3) The Advanced Knee Lifts

*Starting Position*: Start with legs extended straight on the floor, torso propped up on the elbows. In this position people tend to let themselves sag in the chest so keep it high. Shoulders should be kept down.

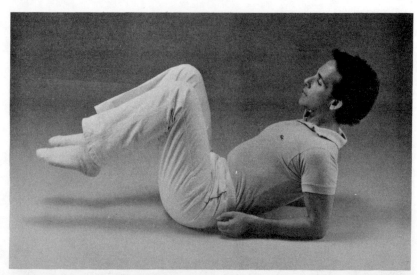

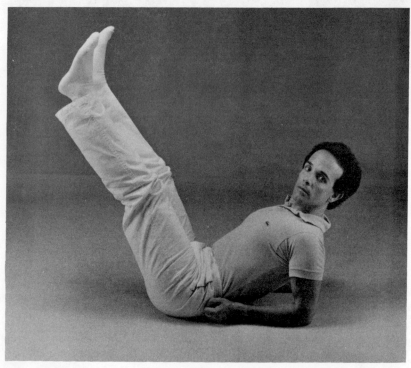

Bring both knees in toward the chest.

Now extend both legs up to the ceiling. Keep thinking of keeping the chest high and the shoulders down. Bend the knees and bring the legs back down to the floor, straightened. Each group of one upward and one forward movement constitutes one repetition.

Start with five repetitions three times, then add five each week.

4) The Torso Lift

With hands behind the neck and chin on the floor, inhale. As you exhale lift the chest off the floor, keeping the legs extended. Do not go up beyond the navel area.

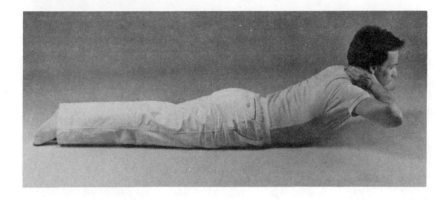

Start with four repetitions three times, then add two each week.

Remember that these exercises should be done as part of your present exercise regime. If you do not exercise regularly you should start with the Daily Rehab Conditioners and the Tension Release Exercises before doing these.

# SUPPLEMENTAL EXERCISES FOR SPECIAL BACK CONDITIONS

*For Prolonged Sitting*

Besides the Tension Relief Exercises that work on the hip flexor muscles, these two simple exercises help to alleviate tension while strengthening the hip area.

1. Sitting in a chair with both feet on the floor place each ankle over the knee of the opposite leg. Do at least ten times on each side a couple of times a day. Try not to move the rest of your body as you lift the leg and cross it.

2. Sitting in a chair with both feet on the floor, lift the knee of one leg in line with its hip joint while twisting the torso in its direction. For example: Lift right knee—twist torso to the right.

3. Sitting in a chair with legs extended, rotate the legs in and out, first bringing the heels together and then the toes. This twisting action will be felt in the hip joint if the legs are kept straight. If you need extra leverage to keep the legs extended, press down with your hands on the sides of the chair's seat.

*For Swayback (Hyperlordosis)*

Most any exercise that promotes abdominal strength and reduces abdominal size will help to correct sway back. Any of the exercises in this book that deal with lower and upper body curls, knee raises, leg extension, will be beneficial if you have a swayback condition. Keep in mind, however, that in most cases swayback is a combination of weak muscle tone and bad mechanical habits. Be sure to read Section Three which deals with body mechanics in general.

### Wall Sliding

This is an old but very beneficial exercise. Stand with your back to the wall, about a foot in front of it. Knees should be slightly bent, feet parallel about shoulder-width apart. Lean your back against the wall. Take a deep breath and exhale, tightening the muscles of the abdomen. You'll feel your lower back get closer to the wall. Hold that position for about twenty counts. Take another deep breath and as you exhale slide down the wall until your thighs are at a 90 degree angle with your torso. Be sure to keep your knees traveling in a direct forward line over the toes.

### For Round Back (Hyperkyphosos)

Kyphosis is normally a curvature of the thoracic area which, when in excess, is called hyperkyphosis and is characterized by rounded shoulders and a sunken chest appearance. Mild forms of this problem respond quite effectively to exercise for better posture, such as those found in Section Three. The following set of exercises should be done slowly using imagined action. As with all exercises involving visualization, read it over a few times before you do it.

#### #1.

1. Sit in a straight-back chair. The top of the chair's back should reach your shoulder blades.

2. Let the chin drop to the chest and let your arms hang loosely at your sides.

3. Take a deep breath and hold it for a couple of seconds; feel the air reach down into your hips. Picture yourself as a flower that has wilted at the base (the lower back) of its stem (the torso). Exhale as slowly as possible. As you do so imagine that, as the air comes up, it passes through the stem, blowing life into it in such a way that the flower straightens.

4. Now follow this image with action. Inhale deeply again. Hold it. As you exhale and the air blows through the "stem," your stomach should tense; the chest expands and pushes the chin up; the shoulder blades relax and the head comes up. Your arms remain at your sides with the shoulders down and back. Hold this position while you breathe evenly, then repeat.

#### #2.

1. Still in the sitting position, keep your torso as straight as possible. Make sure the chest is up and the head is back.

2. Inhale and lift both shoulders to meet your ears.

3. Exhale as slowly as possible. As you do so think of your twelfth rib, the last one down, coming up to meet your chin while your shoulder blades are going down to meet your lower back, which should be pressing at the back of the chair. Breathe evenly in this position. Repeat five times.

**#3.**

1. Sit in between two blocks of wood or two telephone directories. Place your hands in the center of them and press down, lifting your body off the floor. As you maintain the downward pressure you should have a feeling of uplift throughout the spine and chest. Don't let the shoulders sag. This exercise helps to strengthen the lateral muscles of the torso. It will also be beneficial to those with slight scoliosis.

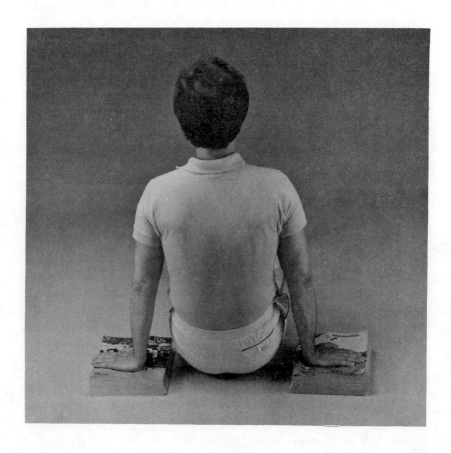

# STRETCHING

The benefits of muscle stretching have been debated among physiologists, anatomists and, surprisingly enough, some physicians. The controversies seem to derive from two main issues: one, that people who engage in stretching do not know enough about it to make it beneficial and end up hurting themselves instead; and two, that there isn't enough medical documentation or informative data to substantiate the benefits that are so widely accepted by dancers and athletes.

Through my own experience I have to agree in part with those who say that most people don't know enough about stretching to reap any benefits from it. In order to properly stretch a muscle or a group of muscles, a person should have a basic knowledge of the muscles he wants to stretch, of the strength or fragility of the joints to which the stretch will apply the most force, of how long to hold a stretch and of how much is enough, or too much. The latter is the killer, for too much forced stretching can render some ligaments unelastic—that is, not able to return to their normal form and thus altering the range of mobility or the form of the joints they protect. Too much stretching can also decrease, rather than increase, muscular suppleness. This is why it's important to know something about your muscles and how to properly stretch *before* you begin.

Muscle fibers can stretch to a little over one and a half times their original length. As they stretch so do, in varying degrees, their connective tissues. Once the applied stress is stopped the fibers and tissues return to their original state. When the stretching of muscles becomes an integral part of a daily exercise routine, as it is in dance, then it is possible to relax the tightness of fascia, to increase muscular suppleness, to strengthen the ligaments that support the joints, and by the combination of all these develop better skeletal alignment. It is this end result that should be one of the major objectives of any fitness plan that relates to back care. Furthermore, when it comes to our backs, proper stretching of muscles opens the spaces between the lumbar vertebrae which is where most back troubles originate, thus relieving nerve compression. Stretching also develops better elasticity in the various ligaments that support our spine. This makes it easier for the back muscles to do their job of stabilization and movement without having to act as supporters as well.

Muscles stretch according to their degree of tone and stretch reflex, which is a property of all functioning muscles that allows them to contract even while being stretched. For those in such professions as dance and gymnastics, where great demands are placed on muscles to perform movements requiring a great deal of coordination, flexibility, balance, precision and control, none of which can be achieved without good postural alignment, a variety of stretching exercises are common practice. Unfortunately, due to the current fitness craze, many of these advanced exercises have been picked up and taught to people whose bodies are not yet ready—and they may never be—to perform such feats. Consequently the body can only react in one fashion—with pain—when it is asked to do something it has not been progressively conditioned to do.

Stretching is usually associated with developing flexibility. But flexibility, as we have seen throughout these chapters, also depends on many other factors. Stretching is more an exercise of the mind than it is of the muscles. In order to stretch you must be able to relax and to do this takes time. Just as you can't expect to stretch a tensed muscle until after it has relieved itself of most of its excess tension, you cannot expect a body to relax until its respiratory and circulatory systems are working at their normal pace and the central nervous system has balanced its commands.

We have discussed the importance of emotional stress and how it is harbored in our muscular system, primarily in the layers and crevices of our backs. We have mentioned that in order to relax we have to train our minds to think positively and to dismiss negative or tension-inducing thoughts. Proper stretching is the ultimate exercise in the combination of mind over muscle. While in everyday movement the mind commands muscle into action, during stretching the mind must take a passive role to allow the muscle fibers to relax and stretch further.

Therefore stretching takes time. When you stretch you cannot have a clock dictating how much time you need to achieve any particular goal unless you are stretching for temporary relief, i.e., getting up in the morning and stretching your arms and yawning. Some days you will be able to reach a certain degree of stretch much sooner than others, depending on various environmental factors that influence our ability to relax: the weather, the place where you stretch, the time of the day all play a role in your mind's ability to let go so that the muscles can follow suit.

Because of the variables that influence how much stretching we can do at a given time, I have divided stretching exercises into two groups: those that provide temporary relief and those that require long-time action. The first group includes those that you can do throughout the day, at any time and practically anywhere. They are designed to give your back fast, but temporary, relief of tension. The long time action stretches are those that should be done as the climax of an exercise regime. Their benefits are long-range and thus can't be seen or felt immediately.

The stretches I have selected for this book can safely be done by anyone, young or old. While the bulk of them are directed to the muscles of the back, others target those muscles in the hip joint and thighs. Whether you are doing the temporary relief stretches or the long action stretches, all of them are fairly easy to do. In fact, chances are you have seen some of them before. But even if you are familiar with an exercise, this book will be most useful if you approach it anew and study the instructions and photographs as though you were learning it for the first time—this way you will be sure of doing the exercise correctly. But first there are some basic guidelines about stretching that you should learn and memorize:

### Stretching Guidelines

1. Stretching is not a contest. If you are stretching in a group never compare what you are doing with what others are doing. Every person has his own individual limits of flexibility.

2. Long-action stretches should only be done *after* a workout. If you've had an aerobic workout you should spend a few minutes bringing your pulse down before doing your stretches.

3. A stretch usually involves the holding of a bodily position for one or more parts of the body, each lasting at least thirty seconds or more. The number of parts being stretched is usually determined by the individual's muscle tone and/or the muscle group being stretched.

4. A good stretch is measured by the way it feels (the ease with which you stretch each progressive time), not necessarily by the added inches or increased angle of flexibility achieved. The "feeling" of a good stretch is developed with time and practice as your mind records and compares present and previous information.

5. Bouncing is a dynamic action which involves contraction and extension. Stretching is a dynamic action which involves continuous extension. *Bouncing tightens while stretching relaxes muscles. Bouncing can injure and tear tendons, ligaments and muscles, but it cannot relax them or make them more flexible.* This is why it is important not to bounce while you stretch.

6. There are three basic stages to a stretch: the natural stage, the working stage, and the overworked stage.

a) The natural stage is determined by the position or angle that your present muscular condition allows you to achieve without effort. This stage is in constant change of increase or decrease. You should spend at least twenty seconds in the natural stage before proceeding to the working stage.

b) The working stage is determined by the amount of residual tension in your muscles during the natural stage, your ability to relax, and the amount of time it takes you to reenact the feeling of your previous working-stage stretch. During the working stage the feeling of stretch must be one of a constant and gradual pulling force, which is felt most strongly on the joints closest to the muscle or muscle group being worked. But this "pull" must not be a feeling of pain, stress or strain. It is the ease of relaxation during the working stage that helps to develop optimum results.

Operating at the working stage is a safety valve of maximum stretch which is controlled by the muscles' stretch reflex. When we try to go over the maximum stretch limit by forced pull or by bouncing, the stretch reflex will activate its contracting mechanism. This will work against the over-stretching of the fibers that could cause possible tear. *Maximum stretch in the working stage can only be achieved by long sustained stretches.*

c) The overworked stage is usually reached when the individual's mind goes from a relaxed state to a competitive state. This state dulls the mind's safety devices and allows the individual to force the muscles and their connective tissues to extreme limits. This is the stage beyond the maximum stretch.

**Four Steps to Proper Breathing While Stretching**

Because breathing is essential to obtain relaxation it is therefore important in learning to stretch properly. In teaching stretching I have found the following breathing-stretching steps easy for most people:

*Step One*: Take a deep breath and as you exhale place your body in the starting position that the stretch calls for. Remember that you should try to take at least twice as long to exhale as you do to inhale.

*Step Two*: Once in that position take a deep breath again and exhale as slowly as you can while clearing your mind of all negative thoughts and concentrating only on your body and on the feeling of your muscles relaxing.

*Step Three*: Inhale again and as you exhale try to reach your working stage. Then stay in that position for a couple of minutes while breathing evenly and never holding your breath.

*Step Four*: Inhale deeply again and as you exhale try to increase the pulling force of the stretch by decreasing the angle between the joints being worked a little more. Then stay in that position for at least thirty seconds. If you are stretching muscles of the limbs or sides of the body repeat the same four steps on the opposite side. It is not necessary to execute a stretch more than one time per session in each position.

With these safety devices in mind and following the four steps to a proper stretch let's take a look at the stretches selected for proper back care.

## BACK TENSION RELIEF FOR THE OFFICE

The following stretch routine is designed to give your back a break from tension. It works on the muscles and ligaments of both the back and hips which can get tight as a result of prolonged sitting. These can be done at any time—the more frequently you do them the better. You'll not only release tension from your back, but will give those muscles some much needed care.

All of these stretches are done with the use of a chair. After a few times you should be able to go through this routine in less than ten minutes. In fact, if you do these exercises instead of having coffee and that donut during your break, you'll lose pounds *and* tension at the same time.

*#1*

Lace your fingers behind you and turn the palms of the hand toward the floor. Try to bring your shoulder blades together by pinning the shoulders back while you look down. Hold that position as you inhale and exhale a couple of times.

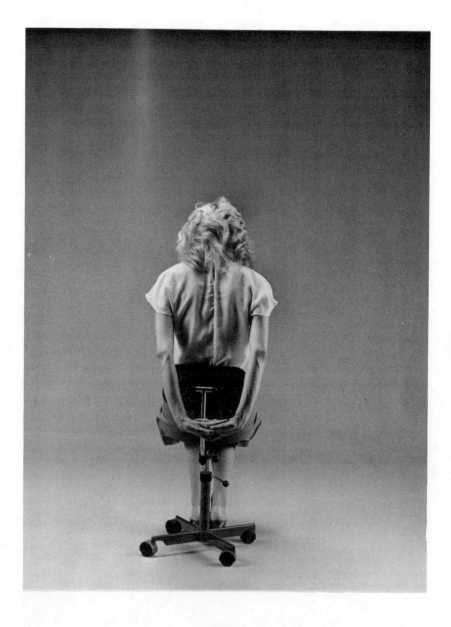

**#2**

Lift both arms and clasp your hands together, crossing the left wrist in front of the right. Let your chin drop down as you reach up as high as you can. Inhale and exhale in that position a couple of times, then change the hand position by crossing the right wrist in front of the left.

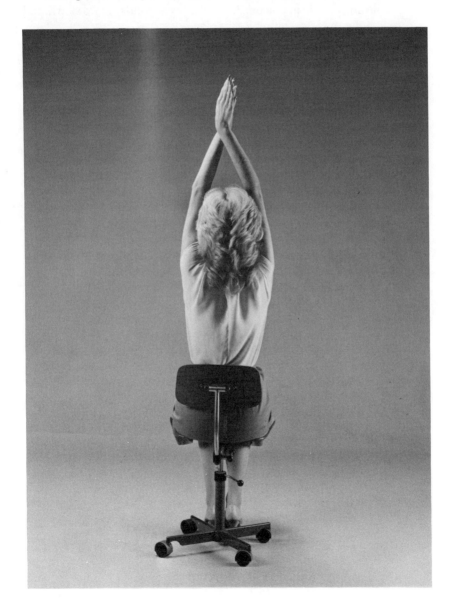

*#3*

Cross the foot of one leg over the thigh of the other and lean over it as if trying to reach the floor. You may feel a pull at either the back of the leg (where it joins the buttocks) of the crossed leg, or in the buttocks, the hip or in all these places. It depends on where you are tightest. Try to inhale and exhale in that position for a few seconds. Sit up slowly and repeat the exercise with the other leg.

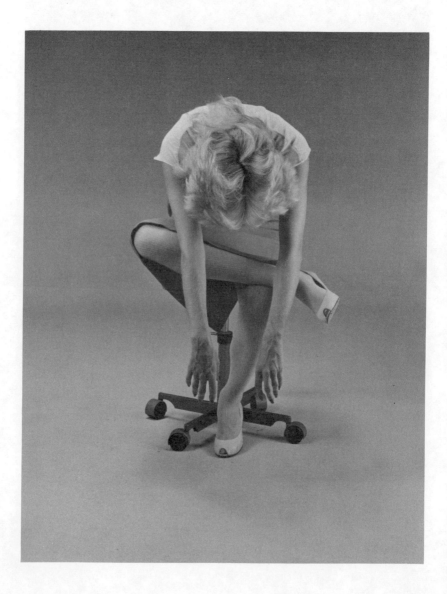

**#4**

With the one thigh crossed over the other, reach down and touch the foot with the arm opposite to the foot on the floor. Extend the free arm over the back of the chair and look away from the feet. Inhale and exhale in that position for a few seconds and change legs.

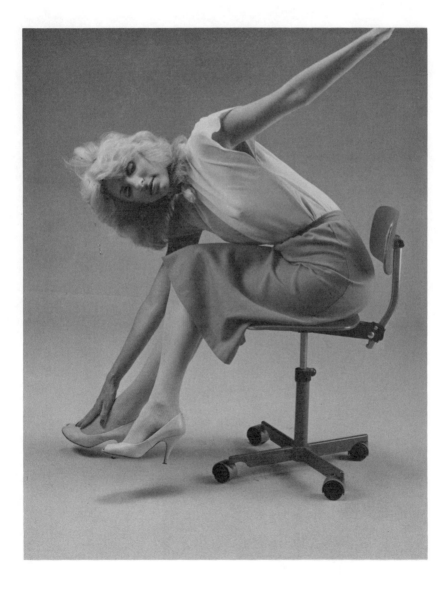

**#5**

Open your feet wide, keeping them parallel. Bend the torso forward so that the chest rests between your thighs. Your head should be down. Place your arms inside the knees and with your hands try to reach around to the *outside* of your feet. Breathe evenly and relax in this position, holding it for as long as you can. Recover from it by rolling up slowly.

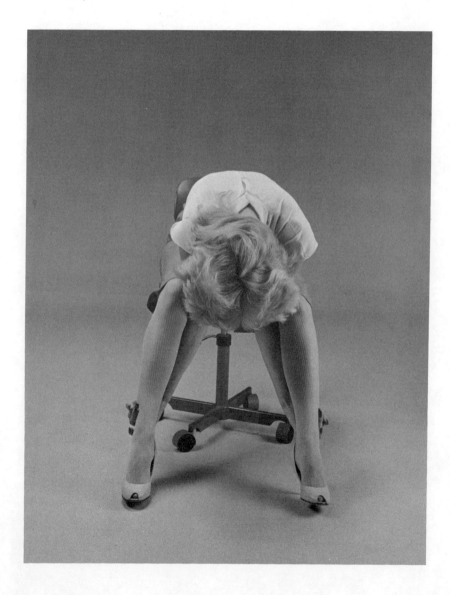

**#6**

Stand behind the chair or with your arms over the edge of a desk. Step away so that you can bend forward without touching your head to the furniture on the way down or up. Bend forward at the hip joint and keep your legs straight.

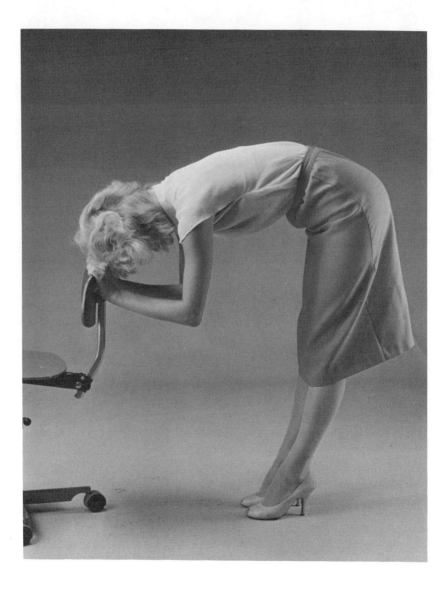

Bend your knees slowly and think of trying to place your buttocks over your heels. Keep the back rounded.

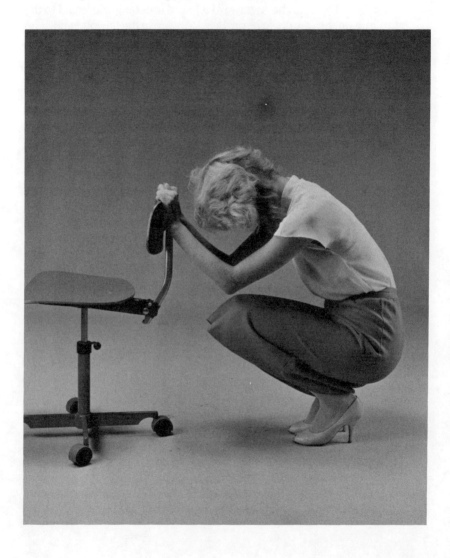

Continue to go down until you're in a squatting position with feet and knees together. Come up slowly, reversing the process.

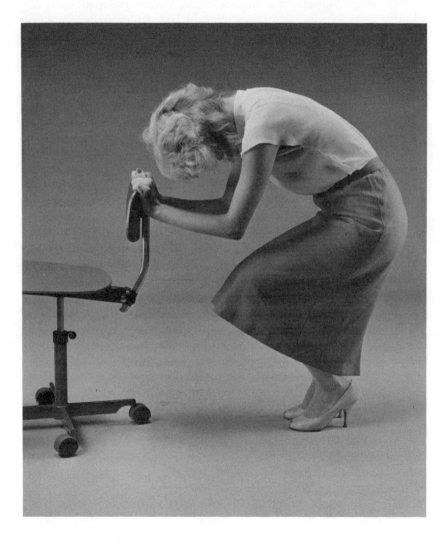

*Reminder:* If you use a chair make sure it is anchored steadily. This exercise has best results if done without shoes.

## LONG-ACTION BACK STRETCHES

These are back stretches that should be used as a supplement to any exercise routine or after any type of rigorous workout. They concentrate on the areas that tend to get tight, such as the back of the legs, hip area, the back and shoulders. Use the four-step procedure described in "Proper Breathing While Stretching" as you go from the natural stage to the working stage. Remember that anxiety has no place in stretching, nor can proper stretching be done while trying to beat the clock. Give yourself ample time.

### #1

Sit on the floor with the soles of your feet together. Hold your feet with your hands. Inhale and exhale a few times, each time thinking of relaxing the back and shoulders and bringing the head closer to the feet. Use your arms to pull yourself toward your feet—gently! Do not bounce.

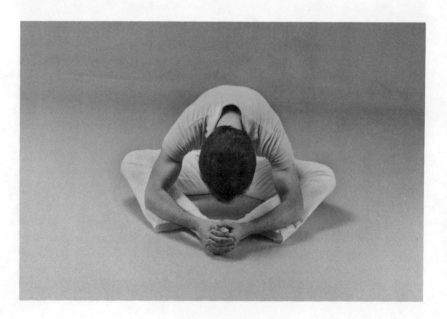

**#2**

*Starting position*: Sit on the floor with knees bent and thighs as close to the chest as possible. Hold your feet with your hands.

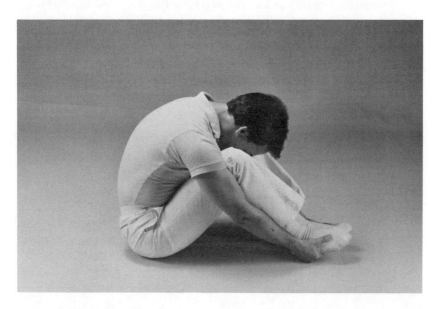

Take a deep breath and as you exhale slide your legs forward. The best way to reach a total stretch as you see in the picture is to apply the four-step procedure and work toward it a little at a time. Don't be

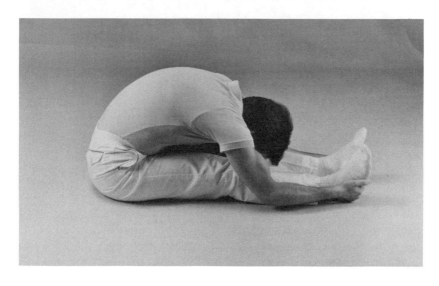

discouraged if you can't place your head close to your knees. This stretch, as do most of the long-action stretches, takes time. But if you do them regularly, within three or four months you will see and feel the difference. Remember that not everyone has the same flexibility. If I don't stretch regularly it takes me a while to reach the position I am showing in the picture.

**#3**

Sit up with legs opened outward, torso straight and hands laced behind the neck.

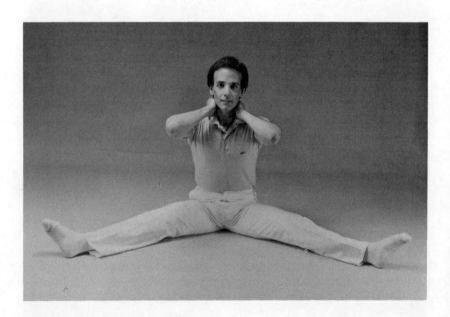

Take a deep breath and as you exhale bend forward as if you were going to place your elbows on the floor. Again, follow the four-step procedure for stretching. Take your time. This stretch will work on the muscles in the back of the legs, the groin and the back.

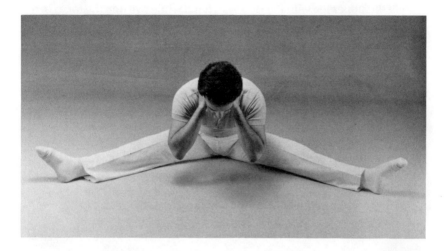

After holding the forward bent position for a few seconds extend the arms forward over the floor. Inhale and exhale slowly, trying to reach forward when you exhale. Concentrate *not on the back muscles but on relaxing the leg muscles*. In no time you will see how far down you can get. Roll up slowly and shake your legs out.

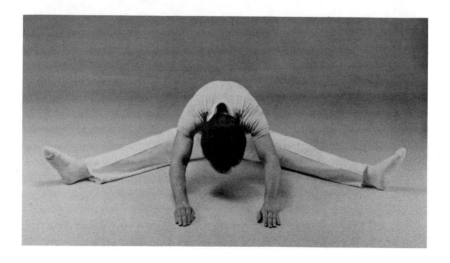

**#4**

Sit up with one leg bent and crossed over the other, as shown. The knee of the leg resting on the floor should also be bent; the foot should be as close to the pelvis as possible. The foot of the upper leg should be placed next to the outside of the knee of the lower leg. Hold the foot of the upper leg with the opposite hand while twisting the torso in the direction of the upper knee. The free arm should be extended behind the body with the hand on the floor for support. Inhale and exhale in this position for a few seconds, concentrating on keeping the torso straight and the stomach tight as you feel the stretch, especially in the buttocks.

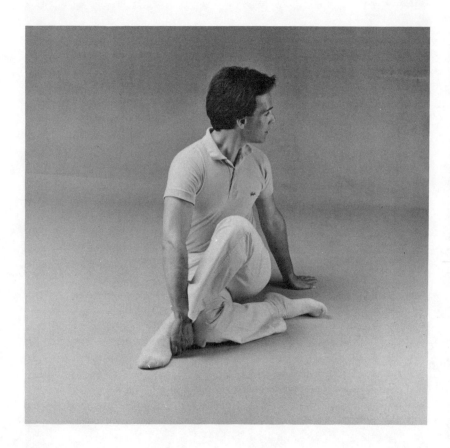

**#5**

One of the easiest and most beneficial of all stretches is the squat. Squat on the floor, letting your knees open outward. Place your hands on the floor between your feet for support. Let the head hang down and feel the stretch in the backs of the legs and throughout the entire back. This is great for tight hip flexors. Spend as much time in this position as possible, then roll up slowly.

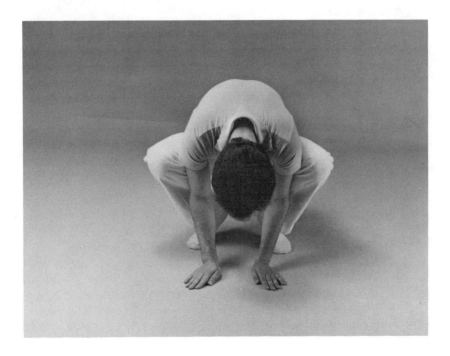

**#6**

This is possibly the most famous of all stretches. It is often given as a test by physicians to determine flexibility of the hip flexors and alignment of the spine. This stretch, though, should never be done before the body has had a good workout and other stretches have been done. There are two ways to do it: The first is by standing with the feet parallel about twelve inches apart. Bend at the hip joint to touch the toes—that's the complete stretch. Although it's simple to do, it is also risky because it's easy to pull ligaments of the spine and the hamstrings and muscles of the legs and back if they're jerked suddenly. That is why you should only do this if you're warmed up with other stretches.

The following approach is my favorite. It takes a little longer, but the results are far better. We will do this stretch in four steps, which should be done following the four-step procedure for stretching.

*Step One*: Stand with your feet parallel, knees bent with your chest resting on your thighs. Keep the head down. Your knees, hips and shoulders should be aligned directly under one another. Place the heels of your hands in front of each foot and press against the floor throughout the entire stretch.

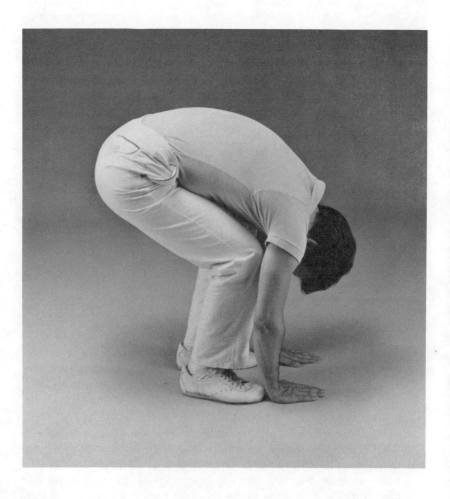

*Step Two*: As you press concentrate on your hip bones. Visualize them rising toward the ceiling, then follow the image with the actual action and begin to straighten your legs. Stop the moment you feel "the pull" on the back of the leg (the hamstring muscles). This is your working stage. Stay there for a couple of minutes. Keep pressing your hands on the floor.

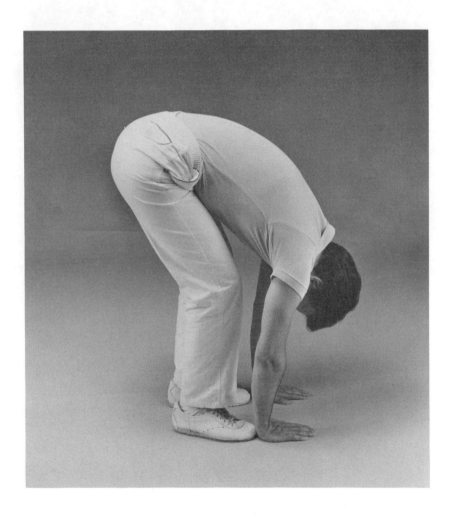

*Steps Three and Four*: Continue to think of the hip bones going directly upward. Follow it again with physical action until your legs are totally straight, as shown. Remember that as the hips rise and the legs straighten the object is to keep the heels of the hands pressing against the floor.

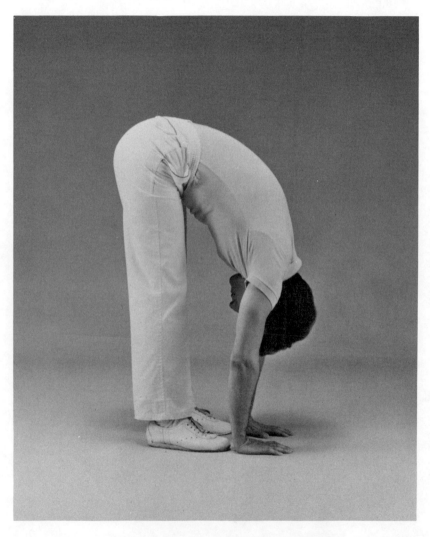

To stand upright after this final stretch, flex the knees again and roll up slowly, as if trying to place each vertebra on top of its lower one a step at a time.

*Note*: It will be helpful if you concentrate more on the hands pressing the floor than on the stretch of the legs and back. By diverting your point of focus you will be able to stretch farther.

### More About the Toe-Touching Stretch

It is a physiological fact that most people have one leg longer than the other. This is analogous to having a dominant right or left hand. Usually the longer leg is the dominant one. Tests have even shown that the majority of us tend to step first with whichever leg is longer, though it is usually the least reliable in terms of weight support.

This difference in length can be the result of several things, one of which is a lateral deviation of the pelvis or of the spine (scoliosis). Such deviation can be caused, as we discussed in Section One, by muscular imbalance—either because of poor muscle tone or because of a person's mechanical habits or habits induced by working requirements. Although manipulation by an osteopathic physician or a chiropractor is often a tremendous help in such deviations when they are due to misalignment of the facets or because of nerve pressure, the toe-touching stretch as outlined above can also be quite successful.

The secret of its success lies not in the achievement of touching the floor with straight legs, but on the slow visualization of trying to keep the hip bones in a horizontal line with the floor as they (the hip bones) rise upward and while pressing the hands against the floor, which helps to equalize the spine and the shoulders.

# SECTION

3

# BODY MECHANICS —CENTERING

Centering is a concept which is introduced to dance students from practically the first lesson. The concept is easy to learn and, when applied, is quite beneficial to back pain sufferers in easing the pain of everyday movement. What it refers to is the imaginary "center" of our bodies, around which our movements should revolve if our posture is correct—that is, if the spine and pelvis are correctly aligned.

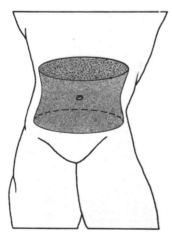

*The center could be thought of as an imaginary drum that sits under the rib cage and above the pelvis.*

Where, then, is the body's center? It can best be described as the body's core, and this is the area of the trunk where we find the muscles that stabilize the head, the neck, the ribs, the spine and the pelvis. To better visualize it think of an imaginary cylindrical structure, like a drum, inside your body. The outer surface would be formed by the muscles of the abdomen, the sides of the body and the muscles of the back. Its lower surface would run parallel with the horizontal plane of the pelvis, above which it would rest. Its upper surface would be located slightly below the

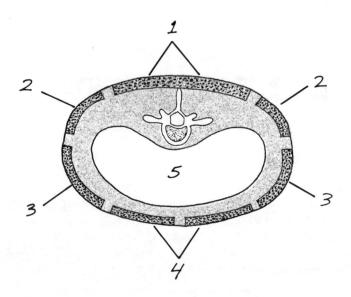

*A transverse section of the superficial muscles of
the center.
1. Spinal muscles: sacrospinalis muscle,
trapezius, psoas major muscle (illiopsosas)
2. Latissimus Dorsi
3. External Obliques
4. Rectus Abdominis
5. Abdominal Cavity*

rib cage. The center of this imaginary drum would be located about two inches below the navel. It also happens that this spot is on a straight line with the body's own center of gravity. Using the navel as a reference point is often helpful to those first becoming familiar with locating the body's center.

You may be wondering if it is really necessary for you to develop an awareness of your body's center. Let me assure you that it is—the center is where all the coordinating and balancing forces of the body come into focus to facilitate proper skeletal alignment, ease of movement without unnecessary energy expenditure, balance and coordination of the muscular system, balanced communication of the nervous central system with the muscular system, and control of all movements, regardless of their simplicity or intricacy. In short, proper body mechanics are not possible without awareness of it.

Although the way in which the body's center relates to overall body mechanics could be a lifetime study, as it is in dance, the study of those concepts that apply to back trouble are few and simple to understand. I have found that when people with a history of back trouble apply these concepts they find them very beneficial in terms of better coordination, less fear of carrying out regular chores and less pain.

Why do we need good body mechanics?

But first, what is meant by body mechanics? Body mechanics refers to the manner in which we carry out movements such as standing, walking, running, sitting, lifting and reaching. While body mechanics describe the way someone moves, good body mechanics describes the quality of that movement.

Good body mechanics are learned and developed throughout our adolescent years. They depend on the role of our parents in our physical activities, our schooling and the sports we participate in, the toys we play with, our musical training or lack of it, our observations of the way our parents and friends move, and our further self-development in a society that for the most part still thinks correct posture and refined movements are too poised for the average taste. And while exercise develops stronger and healthier muscles, it does not necessarily develop good body mechanics. They must be learned. That is the purpose of this chapter.

To learn good body mechanics we must first understand those parts of our physiology that affect them. The central nervous system is the creator and caretaker of our patterns of movements. Therefore, good body mechanics must be achieved by coordination between the central nervous system and the muscular structure. While the brain commands our central nervous system, the center is the place from which good mechanical habits are developed. What do we mean by "mechanical"? Webster's *New Universal Unabridged Dictionary* defines it as "produced or operated by machinery of a mechanism." The body is a machine and as such must be operated according to its design if its performance is to be free of complications. Back pain is the body machine's favorite response to malfunction or misuse.·

The human body is, in a sense, constructed along the same lines as any other mechanical device capable of movement, such as the axle, the wheel, the pulley, etc. The engineering structure which allows movement in different directions is called a lever, and your skeleton is made up of a series of such levers. A lever has a fixed point from which it can move in whatever direction it was designed to move (for example, you can bend your arm at the elbow forward, but not backward). In our bodies our skeletal joints make up the fixed points from which movement is possible.

How close these joints follow the blueprints from which they are designed determine body mechanics—human movement. Of all the different joints in the body and the lines they form, the spine and its various components are the simplest to understand, for all they require is equal balance of pressure and weight from their surrounding pairs of muscles.

A lever must have at least two muscles attached to it in order to move in opposite directions in one plane. Although in theory this may sound complex, the principle is actually simple. The following example will demonstrate the relationship between the body's center, levers, spine, muscles, body mechanics and how they, in turn, may produce pain.

Visualize a seesaw with two people of equal weight at each end of the bar. Because of this equality in weight the bar is in balance; its fixed point is at the center of the bar, and there is equal weight and pressure being applied at both ends. Let's say that one of those individuals suddenly gains ten pounds. What would happen? Obviously, the seesaw would tilt toward his side and would be off-balance. How could it be balanced again? There are only two ways: one, by moving the center on which the bar is resting closer to the heavier side; or two, by assisting the other individual with added pressure to counteract the lack of balance.

Now think of that seesaw as either a vertebra or, better yet, as your spine. The two people at each end would represent the identical pairs of muscle groups that are attached to it. Whenever one side of the seesaw is heavier than the other, force must be exerted on the weak side to restore the balance. In the spine this counterbalancing force comes through the contraction mechanism of the muscles in the back, which surround the center. (In previous chapters we have seen how this unbalanced tone can cause muscle spasm and pain.) But since neither the vertebrae nor the spine can move individually, the first solution, that of moving the center closer to the stronger side, could not apply, or could it? In a sense it can, and that is where the concept of the center comes into play.

Because of the center's location, right above the junction of the spine with the pelvis, its position in relation to movements such as walking, bending or lifting could determine the amount of balance you have when doing these things. Although it is impossible to move the spine as an individual lever to counteract a deficiency of weight and pressure coming from one side, it *is* possible to bring the center closer to a weight-bearing object, as in lifting, and equalize the action on the center's levers.

This example of weight equalization and distribution forms the foundation for the centering suggestions you will find in this section, which will help you achieve better body mechanics and subsequently alleviate as well as prevent lower back pain. Because of the spine's range of mobility, its proper stabilization depends largely on the tone of the muscles that surround the trunk and encase the spine—the muscles of the center.

There are two basic stages to developing good body mechanics. The first is exercise. In Section Two all of the exercises, without exception, are designed for the strengthening of the torso muscles. The second is knowing how to correctly carry out everyday movements, such as bending forward, backward, or sideways at the trunk; bending the knees; walking; shifting weight; and reaching and lifting.

When movements are carried out correctly, they provide the brain with new information which, in time, will render its previously stored information obsolete. The amount of time necessary for this substitution to take place depends entirely on the individual and on whether his newly improved mechanical habits become part of his everyday life or are only used for certain activities. As Dr. Lulu Sweigard states in *Human Movement Potential* (Harper & Row), "A person cannot move successfully by two standards of mechanical quality without paying the price of steady accumulation of muscular strain, perhaps pain, and even impaired movement."

But before we can move, properly or improperly, we must first be able to stabilize ourselves. If we don't we risk being thrown off balance by the movement's own force. The degree to which we stabilize will determine the smoothness of the movement. Again, awareness of your center and proper alignment of the spine over the pelvis and the head over the spine is all-important even before you start.

Assuming that your posture is correct, one of the essentials for further developing better body mechanics is learning to move from the center first and the legs second. Although this concept may seem to dispute the popularly accepted notion of letting your legs do the work, you will see the value of it in regard to back care as we detail the process of proper walking and of stair climbing.

Another premise of good mechanics is based on the physiological fact that muscles are alive even when they're not being used. The thing to do is to use that inner energy in your favor—to control it, not be controlled by it. This is actually more of a brain-nervous system function than a muscular one, and it involves the development of a feeling of movement *before* it is executed. This goes hand-in-hand with the use of imagined action, or thinking before doing, as discussed in Section Two.

One of the most important and often overlooked factors that influences body mechanics is how we *feel* about how we move, as well as our general frame of mind. For example, when we undergo an emotional or stressful experience, it is reflected in our locomotion—depression can cause the shoulders to stoop, while our carriage may improve when we're elated. The mind and body are connected, therefore we *can* consciously improve body mechanics by developing a sense of what is correct posture, what is the correct way of walking with the back properly aligned, etc. Developing a sense of how correct movement feels will also alert us to trouble signals the body sends out—and we'll no longer ignore that slight but persistent ache that might develop in the lower back. In this way developing good body mechanics is also a matter of sensitivity and alertness.

As we've seen, good body mechanics are essential for better back care and health. Implementing them reduces muscular work and strain. They increase the body's devices for safety in response to an outside force or to its own forces. They convey a sense of gracefulness and coordination. Poor mechanics can ultimately render our muscles so inefficient that even a small movement can throw muscles into spasm. Without fault most people who complain to me about backache are those whose knowledge of body mechanics is limited to knowing that they walk with their feet, which in itself is incorrect. We support ourselves with our feet. We walk through the interaction of most of our major muscle groups—a reason why walking is good exercise.

As with exercise, the development of proper body mechanics does not show overnight results, for they depend on the time and thought you put into them. But regardless of age or previous habits, you *can* change the way you move over a period of time. The rewards of such changes will be of longstanding value.

## HOW TO DEVELOP GOOD BODY MECHANICS

Developing good body mechanics is essentially an easy task. In fact its simplicity is its main problem, for preparing oneself for better posture, movement and coordination is not as exciting or challenging as losing those unwanted ten pounds. Even if one day someone unexpectedly comments that you always stand so tall, or look so graceful, it still doesn't have as much effect as if that person were to say you looked younger. The fact is that developing good body mechanics is not a "fun" thing to do, but if you still need some incentive they *will* make you look taller, trimmer, more graceful, healthier and younger.

Aside from the simplicity of it the other common obstacle to adapting better body mechanics is inhibition. Whenever anything relating to changing our pattern of movement comes up, there are always people who will think, "Not possible. I was born with two left feet." Maybe you are one of those people. If so, you needn't worry. What you are about to learn can be done even if you have two right feet—it is that simple.

If you make a conscious effort to practice a couple of movements on your own a few times each day, they will soon become part of your natural way of moving. And although it will take time before these changes become new habits, your back will feel better practically from the start.

### Posture

There is no doubt that most back troubles would cease to exist if people had better posture. But even if you had someone following you around all day reminding you to "stand straight," chances are you still might not stand properly, for the concept of what is proper posture is frequently misjudged. Furthermore, since all of us possess different natural characteristics and body conformations, such a thing as a universally correct posture does not exist. What does exist, however, are concepts on proper standing and moving.

Particularly when it comes to movement, it is easier to learn something new than it is to change something already learned. Therefore, I have formulated some steps that can be easily done by everyone and that will help to improve posture almost immediately. But first it is necessary for anyone willing to improve posture to make an assessment of his or her present postural habits in the standing position. This is done by means of a homemade device that simulates the line of gravity and which, by comparison, can show the individual the types of adjustments needed to balance his or her body according to gravity. But before I tell you how to make such a device I think it is necessary for you to understand the similarities, differences and relationships between the line of gravity, the center and the center of gravity, for all three are essential in the study and development of postural and other mechanical improvements.

LINE AND CENTER OF GRAVITY

The line of gravity is an imaginary vertical line which hangs from the ear and should touch the outer tip of the shoulder and the middle of the hip. Then as it continues downward it travels behind the knee cap and ends up in front of the ankle joint. The line of gravity passes through the center of gravity.

The center of gravity is an imaginary point (as discussed in the section on centering), at which all of its structural component parts balance each other. In the human body in the standing position, it lies in the pelvis, just in front of the upper part of the sacrum.

Proper maintenance of the line of gravity while standing depends on the equality of contraction by the muscles of the back and of the abdomen, which form the circular walls of the center, and on the individual's concept of proper standing.

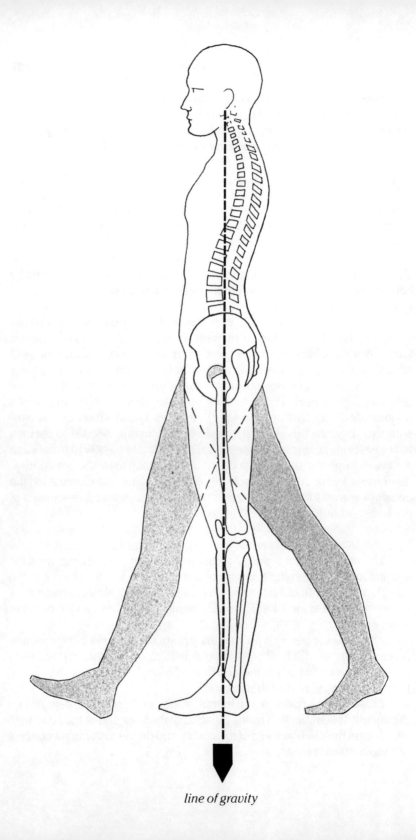

*line of gravity*

Balance is also necessary for correct posture. The body may be considered "balanced" when the weight is distributed in such a way that the body can maintain its own equilibrium without outside assistance. This is possible under the following conditions: a wide base of support; equal distribution of weight around the line of gravity; a line of gravity centered in its base; and weight as close to the base as possible.

All of these principles would be easier to apply if more people had a better understanding of their skeletal framework and its workings. Unfortunately, that is not the case. Therefore, as adults, the easiest and most successful way to straighten our bodies and stand or walk with that balanced look of confidence is through the application of imagined action. Here again we see how our brain determines the way we stand until, through improved images, we condition it to change.

To obtain as close a degree of balance as possible, we must visualize the relationship of the body's largest masses of weight, the head, the rib cage and the pelvis, to the line of gravity. The balance of these structures depends on the manner in which their weight is centered. In my classes I try to teach the relationship of these masses in the standing and walking position by using the image of a spool and needle.

Imagine that your trunk is encased in a sewing spool through the center of which a needle is inserted. The eye of the needle is your head and the spool consists of your rib cage, abdomen and muscles of your back. In other words, the spool is the center. This way all three units are aligned and the center of each part will coincide with the center of all the others.

But posture is not determined only by the trunk's alignment, it is also determined by the trunk's alignment in relation to the pelvis. The center is the area that aligns the trunk with the pelvis. When I speak of posture to my students I also use the image of the pelvis as a champagne glass in which the spool floats. I do realize that going from spools to champagne glasses is rather extreme, but that is what images are all about. What counts is their result and this one works wonders. You'll see.

Having covered the differences between the line of gravity, the center of gravity, and the center, let us now go about the business of determining your postural habits and then see how we can improve on them. First let's assemble the device that will make it possible for you to compare your present posture with the line of gravity.

ASSEMBLING THE LINE OF GRAVITY

1. Take a nail or thumbtack and fasten it in the wall at about six inches above your height.

2. Attach to it a long cord or ribbon. Make sure it touches the floor and has at least two feet to spare.

3. Hang from somewhere in the middle of the cord a paper clip or any small object that will make the line taut, creating a plumb line.

4. With a piece of tape secure the cord on the floor at the spot where it settles. That line represents the line of gravity.

5. Bring the remaining part of the line perpendicularly away from the wall and resting on the floor. Secure its end with another piece of tape. This tail end should be at a 90 degree angle with the wall and in a straight line from the plumb line. Using this device we can now assess your present posture in comparison with the line of gravity, after which you will see how you can achieve correct posture.

DETERMINING PRESENT POSTURAL HABITS

1. Stand barefooted on the segment of the line of gravity that you have taped on the floor. The line should pass right in the front of each ankle, dissecting each foot in half.

2. Feet should be pointing straight ahead and should be parallel. The distance between them should be equal to the distance between your hip

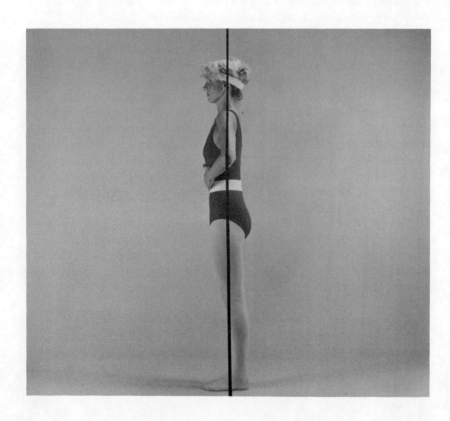

joints. To determine the approximate location of the hip joint, place the heels of the hand over the crests of the hip bone (pelvis) and the fingers over the front of the pelvis pointing down toward the knees. Raise one knee and you will feel an indentation formed by the flexing of the hip in its socket (the hip joint).

3. Put your hands on your waist and bring your elbows in line with the sides of your body.

4. Now that you are in position take a deep breath and exhale, try to relax your stance. The elbow closest to the wall should be pointing at the line on the wall. Look at the line on the wall and see how your body fares in comparison. (This is more easily and accurately done if someone else makes the comparison while you look straight ahead.)

The deviations from the line of gravity that this comparative test can show are many. But there are three extreme ones which specifically increase the opportunity for back trouble:

1. When the upper torso and the center fall backward of the line of gravity.

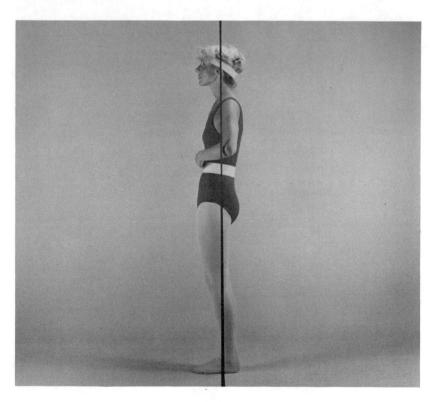

2. When the upper torso and center fall forward of the line of gravity.

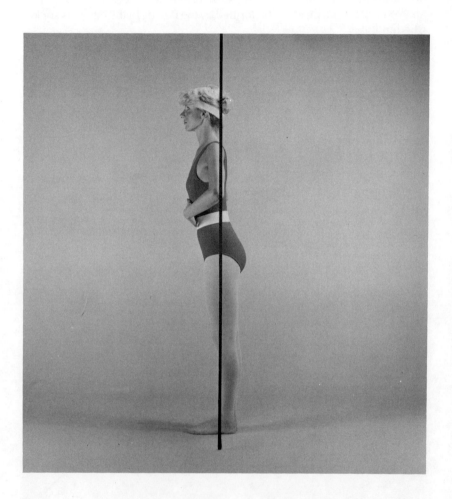

3. When the position of the pelvis is either forcibly or habitually tucked in (tilted too far forward), which often causes the chest to cave in and the shoulders to slouch forward.

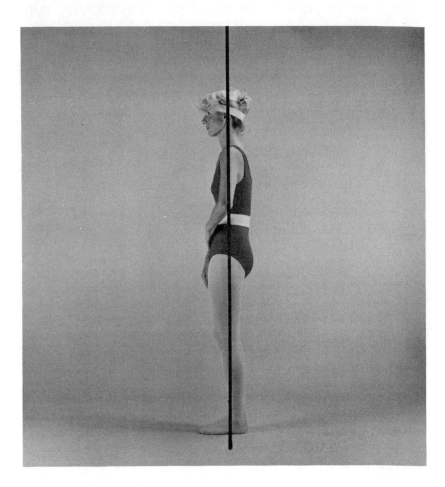

All of these positions have one thing in common: they place tremendous stress on the lumbar curve and can, if persistent with advancing years, lead to very serious conditions such as spondylosis, osteoarthritis and spinal stenosis.

METHOD FOR FINDING CORRECT POSTURE
1. Drop your arms and let them hang naturally along the sides of the body.

2. Without looking down, let your mind search for the spot on your feet where weight is centered. Get a feel for it. If your weight is not slightly in front of the line of gravity, it could be because of the position of your pelvis. Think of the champagne glass image and visualize the glass filled to the rim. Visualize aligning your pelvis by balancing the full glass, then make any physical adjustments that you feel necessary.

3. Now let's work on the top of the body. If you have centered the pelvis correctly, chances are that the trunk will need little adjustment. Think of the spool and needle image. Is the head in the center? Is the base of the spool floating evenly in the champagne glass?

4. Now, without looking down, check again to see if your weight feels centered over the center of the foot. Turn your head to the right and see how much taller and closer to the line of gravity you are.

5. We're not through yet! Let your mind go a step further. Imagine that you are winding thread around that spool, starting from the bottom to the top, close to the eye of the needle. As you visualize that thread winding up and around higher and higher think of it doing the same to your torso. Feel your torso tighten and straighten as the winding continues upward. That feeling of tallness is what you should strive for as often as you can.

Combining imagery with the use of the plumb line will speed up your mind's ability to differentiate wrong from right, especially at first. Once you know how your correct posture feels, you can continue working on developing that balanced feeling without the line, but using the images we've discussed.

Another device that I find successful with my students is what I call Posture Shopping. In this case the image becomes your own reflection. Whenever you go out to do any type of shopping, look at your reflection in a store window before you look at what the store has to offer, checking your posture. Keep doing this from store to store for a block or two. You'll be surprised how soon your postural habits will start changing.

Remember that the moment when you can step on the line, remain still and realize that you are in balance with no or little adjustment is not the end of the exercise. That is just the beginning. Developing good posture has no end. It is a position which is achieved and which must be thought of during the day. Keep in mind that I am not saying you should spend your entire day thinking about posture. The idea is that by knowing the proper way of standing and walking and by practicing it often, our brain will take care of recreating it as it realizes that it takes less work and energy to do it right rather than wrong. But it is up to us to first feed it the right information.

**Proper Standing Position—A Summary**
Before we move on to other aspects of better body mechanics let's

make a last-minute check of the elements necessary for proper standing position. We will start from the feet, going up.

1. Feet should be parallel and pointing straight ahead of the body.

2. The body's weight should be centered in front of the ankles, never on the heels.

3. Each foot should be directly under its corresponding knee and the knee should be lined up directly under its corresponding hip joint (in cases where the knees are turned either inward or arched outward, the line of symmetrical balance should still be a direct line from the feet to the hip joint.).

4. The pelvis should be directly under the trunk. The front of the pelvis should always have a feeling of being lifted, as if it were trying to meet the twelfth rib. It should never feel forcibly tucked under.

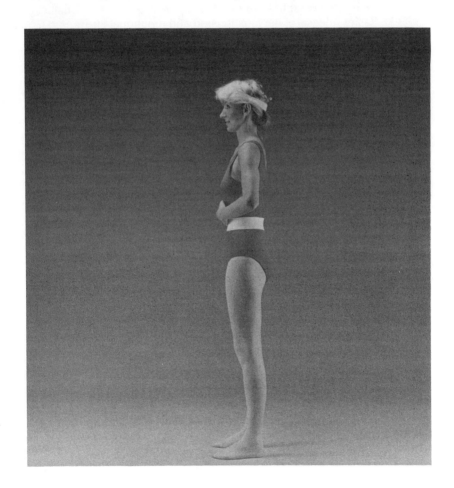

5. The stomach is held firmly in but not forcibly contracted.
6. The shoulder blades feel wider apart and more downward.
7. The shoulders are relaxed and the arms hang loosely alongside the body.
8. The back of the head should be in line with the back of the heels. The head should feel centered over the spine.

### Benefits of Good Posture
1. A trimmer look and better body carriage.
2. Less fatigue from daily activity.
3. More flexibility.
4. Better breathing.
5. Increased safety in movements.
6. Better presence in front of others.
7. Easier release of nervous tension and emotional stress.
8. Better awareness of the start of muscular strain and of what measures to take to prevent it.
9. A stronger and more reliable natural corset.
10. A pain-free back.

### Back Pain and Standing
Although a proper standing position will help to alleviate and even eradicate back pain, a person who must stand for long periods of time should take additional precautions:

1. Never stand for too long with the feet close together. The wider the base you give the trunk, the better.
2. Whether your job requires long hours of standing or household chores such as ironing or cooking, have a small footstool nearby so that you can rest one foot while standing on the other. This helps to reduce muscular strain. Remember that regardless of mechanical balance, all of us have one side stronger than the other (if you are right-handed yours is the right side, etc.). With prolonged standing the weaker side tends to work overtime and this could, in time, promote lateral deviations of the pelvis and the spine. Switch the footstool from side to side periodically.
3. Wearing tight clothes, such as jeans and girdles, minimizes the work of the stomach muscles in maintaining correct posture. If you stand for long periods wear clothes that allow you to move and change stances easily.
4. High-heeled shoes or boots tend to shift the line of gravity and place additional stress on the lumbar curvature. So-called "earth shoes" tend to tighten the Achilles tendon and will also shift the line of gravity. If you have

back pain or a history of it, low-heeled shoes are always recommended.

5. Make a periodic visit to a podiatrist. Although insole supports (orthotics) that help to redistribute and balance your weight properly can be expensive, they will save you money in future medical bills for back care.

6. Do stretching exercises through the day. (See Section Two)

### Shifting

Regardless of direction proper weight change is nothing but transferral of the body's weight from one balanced position (the center of one or both feet) to another while keeping the line of gravity perpendicular to the floor.

While the line of gravity stays relatively the same, the center of gravity changes according to the body's position. In walking the line of gravity must always go from its base, at the center of the foot that is supporting the body's weight, to the center of the traveling foot once the body is over it. In between steps, at mid-stride, the line of gravity goes from the hip joint down to the floor at a spot which ideally should divide the distances between first supporting foot and second supporting foot in equal halves. This means that at mid-stride the body should ideally be balanced between the heel of the front foot and the toes of the back foot.

### Sideward Shifting

From your correct standing position move your center over to the left leg. You will feel the muscles of the leg and thigh contract as they take over the support of the other half of the body's weight. You will also feel a sideways rolling action on the foot you are transferring the weight to. This action will stop the moment that the center of gravity is in line with the inside edge of the supporting foot and the line of gravity is centered over the front of the ankle. In this position the level of both hip bones are still in a horizontal line to the floor although only one of the hip bones has leg support.

### The Wrong Way to Shift Weight

Most people shift weight from side to side by hip movement, or more exactly, by pelvic action. The hip is consciously or unconsciously moved to whatever leg is going to bear the body's weight. Doing this places unbalanced stress on the muscles of one side of the body, besides creating a sideward curve of the spine. Again, shifting weight sideways from one leg to the other should be done by thinking, and then moving, the center as a unit. Although the hip on the weight-bearing side will always be higher than its opposite side, it should never be prominently higher.

### How to Walk Properly—Rolling Action

Proper walking is achieved through a combination of the two previous ways of shifting weight. Let's apply them to the execution of one forward step.

Place the right heel forward and slightly in front of the left foot but do not place any weight on it (just as if you were going to take a step). Your weight is on the left side.

*Step One*: Move the center of the body forward over the supporting left foot until it is felt over the base of the toes (the ball of the foot). Simultaneous to doing this you should have felt that the heel of the right foot starts to dig into the floor as it perceives weight coming in its direction.

*Step Two*: Continue to move the center forward until you feel that you are practically standing between the heel of the front foot (right) and the ball of the back foot (left). In this mid-stride position the line and the center of gravity are directly between both feet and perpendicular to the floor. (It is in this position that the image of balancing the glass of champagne helps to keep the pelvis, and thus the line of gravity, in balanced proportion between the two feet. The mid-stride position is also where bad postural habits and/or skeletal deviations are the most obvious to an observing eye. Swayback is most prominent in this position as the pelvis tends to increase its forward tilt with the swinging of the free leg to take a step.)

By practicing the last two steps you will undoubtedly improve your walk and subsequently lessen back pain. But reading it and doing it once will not do the trick. Only practice makes perfect.

### Turning Movements

Any movement that requires a change from the straightforward pattern of walking or sideways shifting uses the same principles as already stated with the addition of increased work by the center. This is clearly shown by the fact that mechanically *you should always take a step in the direction your body is facing*. And when we speak of "body facing" we are not speaking of where your eyes are looking but of the direction in which the trunk is pointing; it's almost as if your eyes were in your stomach.

I tell my students that, just as a steering wheel determines a car's directional changes, so should our shoulders. They are our body's steering wheel. When turning our bodies the principles of good mechanics to follow are:

1. First turn the shoulders in the direction you want to go.

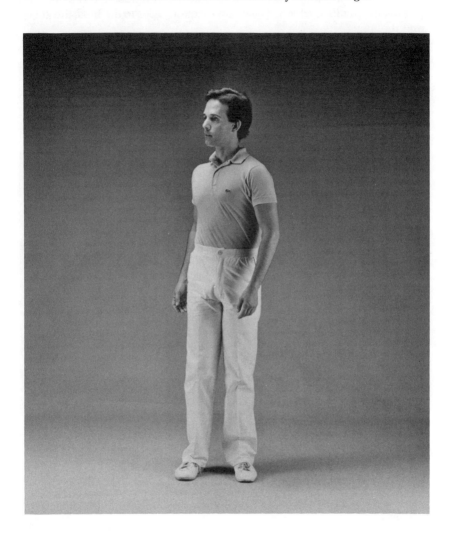

2. Next bring the center in line with the shoulders. This starts the turning mechanism which, as a chain reaction, goes to the hips, the knees and the feet.

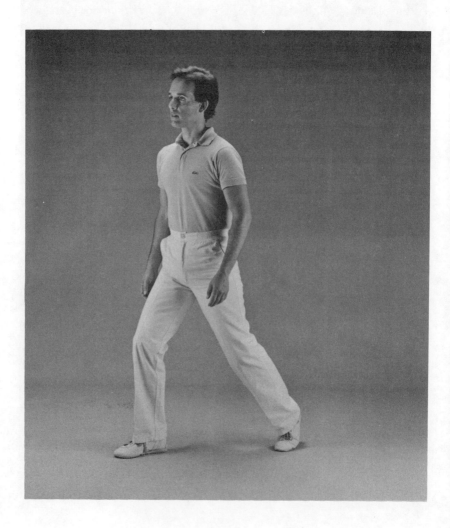

Whenever a twisting or turning of the trunk is needed the hips should move in the direction of the force and the knees should be relaxed, never locked. If you now have back pain, the following suggestion will make things like reaching for an object, opening a refrigerator door, even turning to talk to someone much easier and less painful: Turn the shoulders in whatever direction the objects you want to reach is, or the place you want to go, then let the arms extend and follow in that direction or allow the feet to roll in the direction determined by the shoulders. Beginning your movements in this way will help prevent too much unbalanced twisting of the spine.

### More on Proper Walking Mechanics During Back Pain

1. Keep your steps short.
2. Feet should always be pointing straight ahead.
3. Walk as if two narrow walls, one on either side of you, were rubbing against both hip bones.
4. Make sure your knees and hips are always in a direct line over the feet.
5. Think of your feet as wheels, rather than as flat surfaces. This will help you to walk with a rolling motion instead of flat-footedly.
6. Wear shoes that give your ankles support. During back pain tennis or running shoes that have an arch support are recommended.
7. Remember not to twist the trunk, but to change direction by first turning the shoulders and allowing the body to follow.

## RELIEVING BACK PAIN IN EVERYDAY MOVEMENTS

If you are in extreme pain and are looking for further relief in executing everyday movements or are just getting over a bout of back pain and are fearful of it returning, the following suggestions will help you to execute necessary daily movements such as sitting, bending, climbing stairs and so on, without risking further injury. These suggestions can also be useful for the elderly or anyone who needs help in getting around because of a physical condition.

### Flexing

Proper flexing, or bending, of the body should be done by the cooperative action of the knee joint and the hip joint. Unfortunately, most people bend at the waist which, if you're experiencing back pain, is the last place you should bend. Bending actions are involved in sitting, lifting, stooping, reaching, etc. All of them follow the same rules of mechanics, whether bending takes place just at the knees, the hip joint or both.

### Knee Bending

A knee should always bend in the direction its foot is pointing. The deeper the bending action the farther forward the knee should travel over

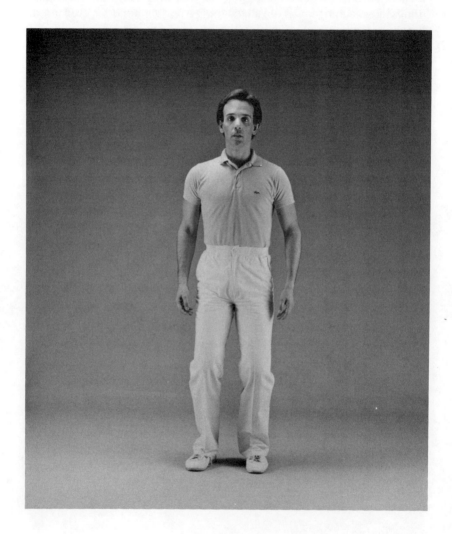

the toes' line of direction. Feet should either be parallel as in the proper standing position, or in a semistepping position. When your knees bend the trunk should be kept steady with a feeling of uplift as it goes down. The buttocks should feel as if they were going down on a direct line to meet the heels.

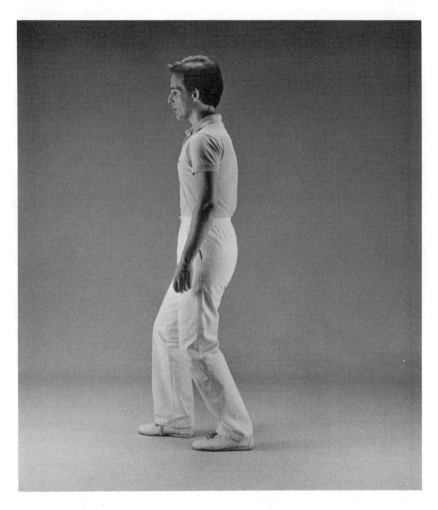

There comes a point in this bending action when the buttocks can't continue downward and must be diverted backward. This point is determined by the flexibility of the hip and knee joints and the muscles of the thighs. When this point is reached then the trunk starts its flexing action over the thighs. Never let the knees sway outward or inward while bending.

This places too much stress on the ankle, knee and hip joints. It could cause further loss of balance and additional back pain.

### Flexing of The Trunk

Bending of the trunk should always take place at the hip joint and the spine should be kept straight until the trunk reaches a 45 degree angle (in forward bending) with the thighs. If the thigh joints are not flexible even this angle will be hard to reach without putting stress on the back. Backward bending of the spine is seldom done in everyday movement and should be especially avoided during a painful condition. Once this subsides, however, the individual should look into exercises which, through hyper-extension (back bend) movements, the muscles of the back can be strengthened. Anytime the trunk is bent forward or backward, the knees should be kept bent and the feet again in stepping position with the knees directly over them. Again, remember that the wider the base the easier and safer it is for bending actions to occur.

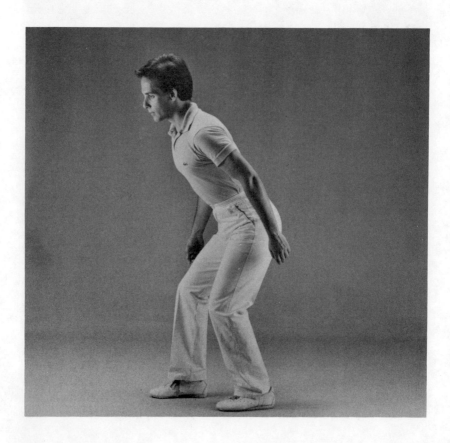

**Our Arms**

Many people who experience their first attack of back pain do so immediately or soon after engaging in manual work. The problem lies in the fact that we think of most types of movements that involve the arms as manual, meaning hands. In actuality, such movements mainly involve the arms. Remember that the way in which we perceive a movement in our mind determines the manner in which we execute it. And in body mechanics, the manner in which we execute movement is everything, which is why it's important to note this distinction.

For most people the use of the arms is associated with strength or power. Our limbs are extensions of the body's center, and it is from their attachment to the center that the real power of the arms flows. The arms themselves have few muscles to develop; it is primarily in the shoulder and upper back region that the strength and power originate. In fact, of all the muscles of the arms only one, the biceps, can develop the kind of strength found in the upper back. And even then, the biceps have nothing to do with the strength of the arms; its job is to flex the elbow and rotate the hand. Nevertheless, this muscle gets more attention than most others.

In order to develop better mechanics with our arms we must change our point of focus from the two most seemingly obvious components of the arm, the hand and the elbow, to the shoulders and the shoulder blades.

As we've seen, most daily movements are executed by habitual reproduction. In order to change a particular movement we must change the original "file" of how we repeatedly do something. Visualization or imagined action is, again, the easiest way to do this.

Let's try this simple experiment which will help you to see and feel the difference between doing a movement by habitual reproduction and by applying imagined action and changing the mechanics of it.

Place a small object, one that you can easily grasp, on a table in front of you. Place either your right or left hand on your thigh. Look at the object for a minute and reach for it. What do you see? You will of course see your hand going for it. What did you feel? You felt the object the moment your hand touched it, right? Okay, now put the object back on the table and your hand on your thigh. Look at the object and in your mind picture a straight line that goes from the back of your shoulder blades to the object. Close your eyes and keep thinking of that line. Visualize how each part of your arm, starting from the shoulder down, will follow that imaginary straight line, section by section: upper arm first, then the elbow, lower arm and hand. With eyes still closed reach for the object. Feel the force of the movement coming from the shoulder blades like a current of electricity that slowly brings the arm in line with that straight imaginary line you had pictured, until you feel the object in your hand. This time you should have felt all parts of your arm in motion, beginning in the shoulder area. The last thing you felt, not the first, was the object in your hand.

What you have just done in this experiment is given your brain new information about a movement you have done many times before. Because we're creatures of habit, it will take several repetitions using imagined action before the mechanics of that movement will become an integral part of the brain's file.

### Sitting

1. Take a step back so that your leg touches the edge of the chair. Although this may sound like a minor point, it's an important one, since it gives your body the wide base it needs from which to move. Bend the trunk forward at the hips. Your knees will automatically flex, or bend.

2. Aim the buttocks toward the angle created by the seat and the back of the chair.

3. If you have been in bed for some time, don't hesitate to use the arms of the chair to help you. As you sit back either place your hands on the arms of the chair, or, if there aren't any, place your hands on the side edge of the seat of the chair and ease yourself down.

4. The same image given for proper walking, that of walking between two narrow walls that rub against the hip bones, should be used when sitting down. This will avoid wobblying of the trunk or tilting of the pelvis as you sit.

TO GET UP FROM A SITTING POSITION:

1. Place your feet in a stepping position.

2. Bend forward at the thigh joints, not the waist.

3. Keep your weight centered over the feet as you press down on the floor and the trunk of the body reaches its upright position.

4. Use the image of the narrow walls to retain your balance as you get up.

### Pushing or Pulling Objects

1. Brace your legs in a position that gives your trunk a wide base. This is best done by standing at about one and a half arm's length from the object and then taking a step toward it.

2. Make sure the knees are aligned over the feet so that when they must bend they will do so over the feet's line of movement.

3. Adjust your own center of gravity to that of the object. If the object's is lower than yours, bend the knees to compensate for it. Never try to push or pull an object whose center of gravity is above your chest level.

4. If possible push with your hands at about shoulder-width apart and

at chest level. In applying pressure to push do so by bending the trunk (at the thigh joint) and letting the forward force be transmitted through the arms from the legs. Never use arm force alone. This will only put stress on the back and could cause the lower back to bend backward, producing a spasmodic reaction in the small muscles of the back. When pulling an object toward you, bring your trunk as close to the object as possible and, using the trunk as a lever from the thighs, pull the object toward you. In both pushing and pulling the arms are just a means of support and grip. It is the trunk and the center's muscles that should do the work.

### Reaching Upward for an Object

1. Stand far enough away so that you can take a step toward the object.

2. Imagine a straight line from your shoulder blades to it.

3. Your trunk and arms should be inclined forward over the thigh of the step that was taken.

4. If the object is heavy bring it down to your body (as close to your center as possible) first before placing it on a surface.

5. Taking a heavy object from a shelf to a lower surface without first bringing it to the body can trigger some pain, especially in a weak back. The same can happen if you stand too close to the object. The weight of it could cause your arms to swing back over your head provoking a certain degree of hyperextension from the trunk (back bend), which could also place pressure on the lower back muscles.

### Picking Up an Object from the Floor

1. Keep in mind what is basic to good body mechanics: knees flexed with feet in a stepping position so as not to put undue stress on the back, and bending *from the hip joint*. If you are right-handed, stand with your left foot next to the object. This allows more room for forward bending.

2. If you must bend sideways to pick up the object, remember that your control depends on the muscles on the far side of your body from the object. Never drop one side of the body to pick anything up. Think long and extended.

3. Never try to pick up anything with the knees locked or with feet side by side while bending forward from the trunk. To do so will put stress on the knees, which are the weakest of all joints.

### Lifting a Heavy Object

1. Don't ever attempt to lift a heavy object without first sizing it up. Consider which part of it you can get the best grip on. Get an idea of the object's center of gravity.

2. Before you pick it up first visualize the steps you are going to take:

a. Take a step toward the object in order to widen your standing base.
b. Lower your body by first flexing the knees, then the trunk at the thigh joints.
c. Place your hands on the object and concentrate on keeping the stomach firm. Take a deep breath.
d. Exhale as you bring the object over your thighs and close to your center.
e. Take another deep breath and as you exhale start straightening your legs without moving the object.
f. Finally use the momentum of the legs to straighten the trunk and bring your pelvis (your own center of gravity) under the object or as close to it as possible.

### Carrying an Object

While the manner in which you carry an object is determined by its size and weight, there are some general rules for back safety that apply to almost everything:

1. Carry the object as close to your center as possible.

2. The trunk should always be kept as straight as possible and the center's muscles should be held firm.

3. If you're carrying the object with a suspended arm, concentrate on keeping the lateral muscles of the body on the side closest to the object tall and elongated. The more heavily a force pulls you down, the more you should pull up to balance and counteract such force.

4. If you must carry a lot of weight over a distance and cannot use a backpack to do so, then hold the weight with both arms close to the center's muscles. Keep your knees slightly bent and allow the trunk to bend forward at the thigh joints so that most of the extra weight is felt by the thigh muscles.

5. If your pelvis has a lateral deviation (one hip higher than the other) it is best for you to carry an object, like a shopping bag or attache case, on the side opposite to your lateral prominence, not on the tilted side. This may also feel more comfortable.

6. If you carry objects by shoulder straps it is recommended that you constantly change sides and not get used to just one side.

### Climbing Stairs

1. Place the whole foot, not just the ball of it, on the higher step.

2. Move the trunk (at the thigh joint) forward over the thigh of the higher leg.

3. Press down on the step with your foot and bring your center over the bent knee as you lift the torso over the thigh.

4. If you have acute pain and must climb stairs do so as previously directed but place a hand over the bent thigh and press down on it as the torso lifts up.

### Going Downstairs

1. Never step on a flat foot. Always try pointing the feet so that the toes feel the step first.

2. If the steps are too steep to do this, go down sideways and hold on to a rail or the wall for support. This is also the best way to go down steps if you have acute back pain.

### Back Pain and Sleeping Habits

I don't know of anything that is more difficult to do than to change one's sleeping habits. But the fact is that many back conditions have been traced to sleeping habits that changed the alignment of a person's spine over a period of years.

Earlier on we spoke of the two best sleeping positions during back pain: the V sitting position and the fetal position. The latter is the easiest to sleep in and is best for your back. The worst position that you can sleep in is lying on your back or face down with legs extended, as this will only pull your pelvis down even more and your back will feel the effects sooner or later.

If you sleep on your side make sure that you use a pillow, never your arm, on the side of your head. Otherwise your head will be thrown out of alignment with your spine. Sleeping consistently with your head on your arm can also cause tightness in the shoulder blades.

One commonly accepted fact is that the mattress you sleep on should not be so soft that it adjusts to the contours of the body. Although this is the general rule there are always exceptions; I have also heard of people whose back pain ended the day they assembled their water bed.

### Back Pain and Sex

Abstention from sex during a bout of back pain is not necessary unless the pain is so acute that it is immobilizing. Otherwise, it just takes a little ingenuity and cooperation between partners. It also requires that the affected person take a less aggressive role. Although low back constriction during sex can cause back pain, contraction of the buttocks and comfortable forward movement of the pelvic structure is one of the most basic exercises recommended for rehabilitation in back pain. The emotional release that accompanies lovemaking also serves to relax the muscles of the back. In this sense, the sex act can be superb exercise for those suffering with low back pain.

There are a number of positions that can be used by both partners which make penetration easier and minimize the role of the back muscles. The most favored ones are with both partners lying on their sides facing each other, or lying on their sides facing in the same direction with the man approaching insertion from the back (called the spoon position), or the sit-up position, where one person sits inside the embrace of another.

# THE SPORTING BACK

Nowadays you can't help but to be constantly reminded to exercise; it is one of the advertising media's best hooks. One of the most popular ways of exercising today is, of course, jogging, which people have taken to like bees to honey. Unfortunately, most people begin without a medical examination or adequate preparation. In fact, most people running today are people who haven't previously exercised. They hope that jogging will be a catch-all form of exercise that will not only maintain cardiovascular fitness, but will result in a trimmer body as well as provide a release from daily tensions. This can only be achieved when the mind and body work together. This means that when you go out jogging, you must try to concentrate on what you are doing and at the same time release all other thoughts that could cause stress. If you fail to do this you will only be adding tension onto the tension your muscles are already creating by jogging.

People with back trouble especially should not jog without first seeing their doctor. Furthermore, people whose back trouble is closely related to bad postural habits could hurt themselves further by jogging unless they are constantly aware of their posture and the proper mechanics involved in jogging.

Recently, while taping an interview for the television show *Real People*, Byron Allen, the host of the show, and I went to New York's Central Park Reservoir. This is a place where one can find people jogging at all times of the day. I was amazed to see the number of people who would lean against a tree and do what they thought were muscle stretching exercises prior to their running. Although their intentions were good, nine out of ten were far from stretching adequately before they quit. Many, in fact, were not executing the stretches properly, but were simply pulling their back and leg muscles. As we've learned in the section on stretching, this only tenses the muscles more. Muscles pull the body to work, but they do not react well to the body pulling on them so erratically. Doing this only causes the tendons to fight with rigidity, and overall flexibility of the joints is decreased.

To help those of you who are joggers or weekend athletes with weak backs, I've included a closing chapter of stretching exercises to be done both before and after running or working out.

*Note*: Remember that these are stretches intended to gradually prepare your muscles before activity. Each exercise should be done once on each side, using the four-step procedure for stretching.

### WARM-UP EXERCISES FOR THE WEEKEND ATHLETE

*#1*

*Step One*: Stand in a stepping position with your weight over the front leg. Place the toe of the back leg on the floor and hold your arms in front of you with fingers laced, palms turned forward.

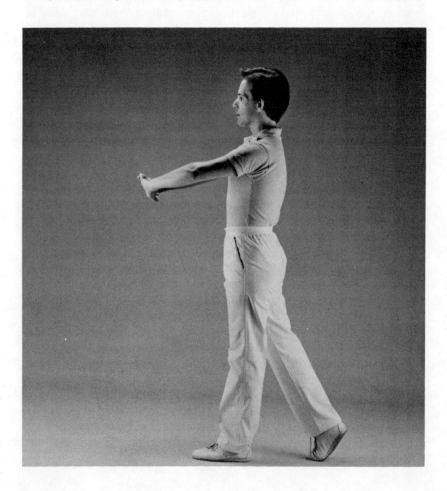

*Step Two*: Inhale and as you exhale stretch upward with the arms while bending the weight-supporting knee. Try to place the back heel on the floor. Your weight must be kept forward throughout. This stretch works on the back of the leg, the Achilles tendon, the hamstrings, the quadriceps of the front leg and the muscles of the upper and lower back.

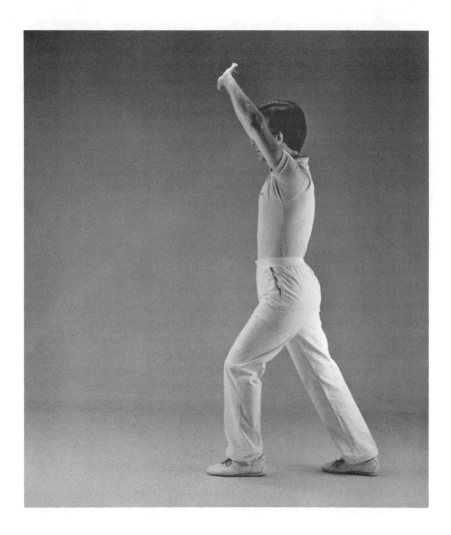

**#2**

This should be done while holding onto something for support. While in a standing position bend the knee and grasp the leg at the ankle; now try to bring it toward the buttocks. Notice in the photo that the bent leg should be slightly in front of the straight supporting leg. This allows stretching of the thigh muscles without increasing the curve of the lower back.

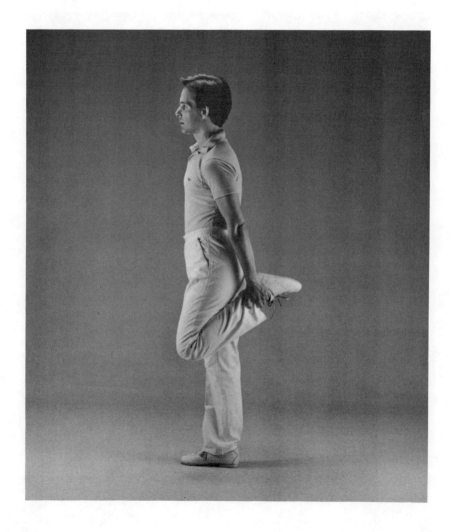

**#3**

As shown, take a large step to the side and slightly forward from the other leg. Bend the forward knee (making sure it bends directly over and in the direction the toe is pointing). At the same time turn your

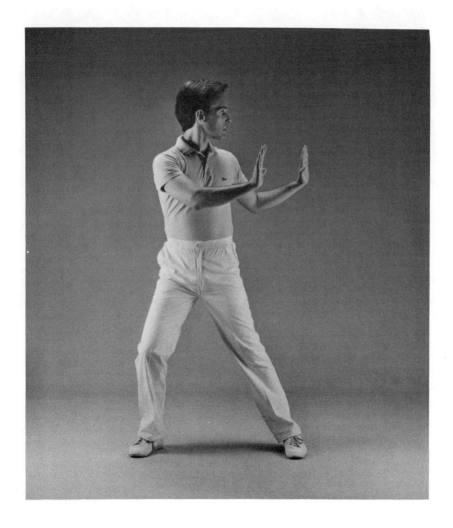

torso toward the straight leg. Do so slowly, twisting as far as you can. It is important to note that as you twist there should be no movement in your hips at all. They should remain facing forward. You should feel the stretch in your thighs as you twist and your weight shifts to the front leg.

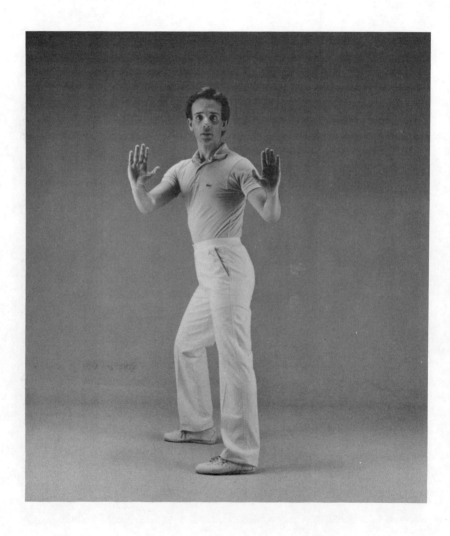

**#4**

*Step One*: As shown bend at the waist and lean forward so that your hands and feet are firmly planted on the floor. Put enough distance between them so that your legs and back are straight. Arms should be in a direct line with the torso.

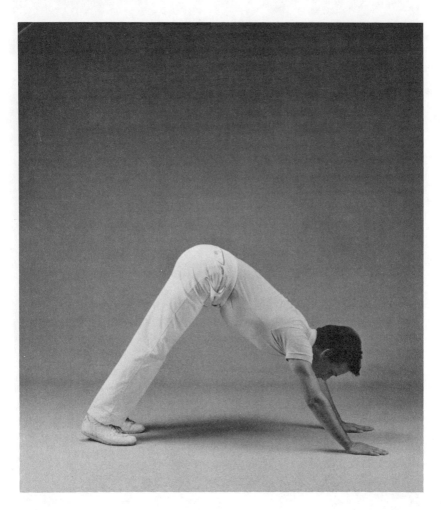

*Step Two*: Alternate pressing one foot at a time against the floor until its heel rises. The heel of the other foot should lower simultaneously. This is a good stretch for the hamstring muscles. Do it slowly, staying in each position for a few seconds.

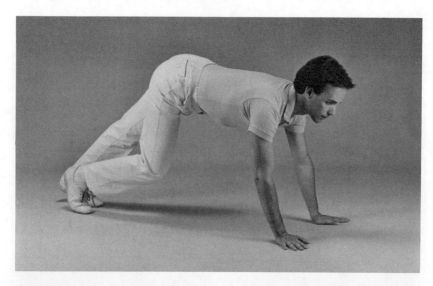

*Step Three*: With both legs straight, try to walk your hands back to a toe-touching position, moving one hand at a time.

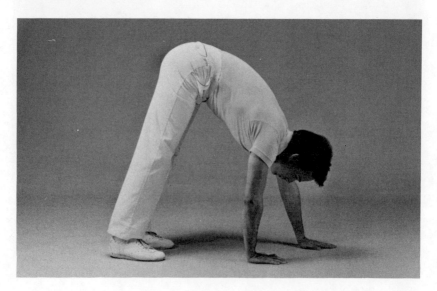

**#5**

*Step One*: Lunge forward with one knee bent, as shown. Try to keep the chest over the bent knee and the hands on the floor directly under the shoulders. The back leg should be straight and the head down with the hips high. Inhale.

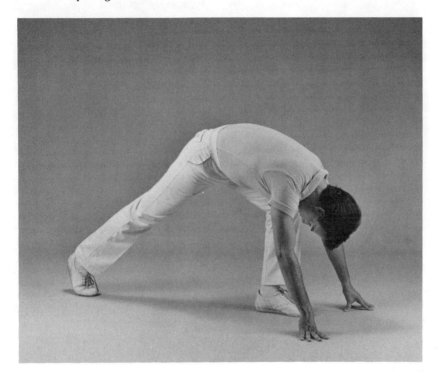

*Step Two*: Look up as you exhale. Let the bent knee flex further and allow the hips to drop to the floor. Stay in this position for a few seconds. You'll feel the stretch mainly in the thigh muscles.

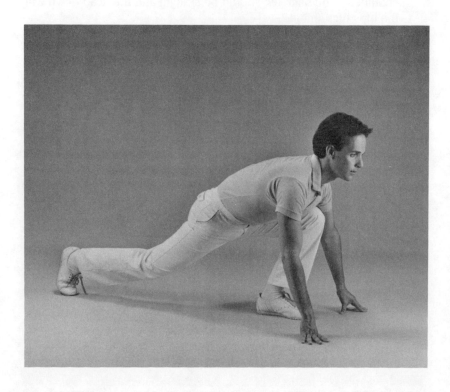

# AFTERWORD

After completing THE BACK BOOK I wondered if there was anything I'd left out—possibly some recent development that I was unaware of as I wrote it. Frankly, I was hoping for something spectacular that would benefit many back pain sufferers. I called Dr. Paul Scoles, an orthopedic surgeon at New York's St. Vincent's Hospital, who has been a great help to me in writing my books. I asked him if there were any new developments I should make my readers aware of, or one last piece of advice I could leave them with. To my surprise he said he had just the thing—a miracle cure which he gave to all of his patients. My heartbeat quickened. I could already see millions of people being helped by his final words of advice . . .

"Lose weight. Exercise regularly and stand up straight." That was the "miracle cure" he promised me. Needless to say, I was disappointed, but not for long. I realized, of course, that there is no such thing as a miracle cure for anything, but I was encouraged that his advice is the same message I've tried to get across in this book. Therefore I will use his words as the basis for *my* final words.

If you are overweight statistics show that the chance of your someday having back problems is quite high. The latest report issued by the National Society of Actuaries indicates that slender people live longer. If you are overweight you should lose weight not just to prevent back problems, but for your general health. Studies also show that weight loss must be a combination of lowering the caloric intake *and* exercise. In an article published in the New York *Times*, August 3, 1983, health and science writer Jane Brody wrote, "Without exercise, the new findings show nearly all attempts to lose weight and keep it off are doomed from the first spoonful of cottage cheese."

People today still think of exercise in terms of reaching short-range goals—an upcoming wedding, bathing suit weather—and not as an integral part of their weekly routine. Most people, especially women, will do it to look better rather than to feel better, and when they reach their desired weight they tend to decrease their exercise routine or stop altogether.

Why is that? I believe there are two reasons: one is that the older we get the lazier we get, and two is that, as I mentioned earlier, exercise is boring.

**189**

So, too, is getting up at 6:30 every morning and traveling to work so we can pay for food, rent, vacation and doctor's bills, the latter of which would be considerably less if we kept fit. But we do it because we have to, and so it should also be with exercise.

People with back pain have additional reasons for shying away from exercise because they fear they will do something to hurt themselves even more. As I've tried to point out in this book, this is a well-founded concern. Remember, however, that these exercises are rehabilitative only—they're not meant to make you the sex symbol of the neighborhood. The goal is to get you to a position from which you may begin a more rigorous exercise program without fear. Once you've completed the four week routine of Daily Rehab Conditioners, you should continue to do those exercises, but add to them some of the supplemental ones found in this book or exercises from some other source. But you must *continue* to exercise if you're going to maintain a strong, healthy back.

As far as the last part of Dr. Scoles's advice is concerned, relating to standing up straight, I think I've made my point as much as possible regarding posture. Nevertheless, I will add one last word of advice.

Unless you can afford to have a physical therapist with you for twenty-four hours a day, no one but you can make improvements in the way you stand and move. It takes discipline and determination, but it *can* be done. It is said that we are the masters of our own destiny. Although I don't buy that entirely, I do believe that our bodies are part of God's gift to us and it is our responsibility to care for them as best as we know how.

A healthy body, free of back pain and undue stress is a body that has been carefully directed along the paths of proper nutrition, exercise and daily care. I hope that each of you will apply the principles outlined in this book so that your back will be as healthy as it should and can be.

# BIBLIOGRAPHY

HEALTHFUL LIVING: A TEXTBOOK OF PERSONAL AND COMMUNITY HEALTH by Harold S. Diehl, and Willard Dalrymple (McGraw-Hill, 1973)

HARRISON'S PRINCIPLES OF INTERNAL MEDICINE, 8th Ed., Ed. by Thorn et al. (McGraw-Hill, 1976)

YOGA FOR BEAUTY by Michael Volin and Nancy Phelan (Bell Publishing Co.)

THE COMPLETE BOOK OF SPORTS MEDICINE by Richard Dominguez (Scribner, 1979)

REVIEW OF GROSS ANATOMY, 4th Ed., by Ben Pansky (Macmillan, 1979)

THE SLIPPED DISC: RELIEVING AND UNDERSTANDING YOUR BACK TROUBLES by James Cyriax (Herman Publishing, 1975)

THE NEW APPROACH TO LOW BACK PAIN by Arthur Fumeson (Berkley Publishing Corp., 1975)

THE BASIC BACK BOOK by Anne K. Rush (Moon Books, 1979)

BACK PAINS: QUICK RELIEF WITHOUT DRUGS by Howard D. Kirrland (Simon & Schuster, 1981)

BACKACHE, STRESS AND TENSION by Hans Krauss (Simon & Schuster, 1978)

HOW TO CARE FOR YOUR BACK by Hugo Keim (Prentice Hall, 1981)

CLEMENTE'S ANATOMY by Carmine D. Clemente (Lea & Febiger, 1975)

FREEDOM FROM STRESS: A HOLISTIC METHOD by Phil Nuernberger (Himalayan International Institute, 1981)

ANALYSIS OF HUMAN MOTION: A TEXTBOOK IN KINESIOLOGY by M. Gladys Scott (Irvington, 1963)

PHYSIOLOGY OF MOTION by G. B. Duchenne (W. B. Saunders, Philadelphia, 1959)

HUMAN MOVEMENT POTENTIAL: ITS IDEOKINETIC FACILITATION by Lulu E. Sweigard (Harper & Row, 1974)

MUSCLES ALIVE by Basmajian, J. V., 3rd ed. (Williams & Wilkins, Baltimore, 1972)

CLINICAL ELECTROMIOGRAPHY by M. P. Snorts (Williams and Wilkins, Baltimore, 1972)

KINISEOLOGY AND APPLIED ANATOMY; THE SCIENCE OF HUMAN MOVEMENT, 2nd Ed. (Lea and Febiger, Philadelphia, 1963)

READINGS FOR AN INTRODUCTION TO PSYCHOLOGY, 3rd edition, edited by Richard A. King (McGraw-Hill, 1961)

GENERAL PSYCHOLOGY by Edgar Vinache (American Book Co., 1968)

HANDBOOK OF EXPERIMENTAL PSYCHOLOGY by S. S. Stevens (John Wiley and Sons, 1951)

THE THINKING BODY: A STUDY OF BALANCING FORCES OF DYNAMIC MAN by Mabel E. Todd (Dance Horizons Inc., 1968)

*"Electromyographic Studies of the Role of the Abdominal Muscles,"* by M. J. Walters, American Journal of Physical Medicine, 1957

*"Electromyographic Studies of Postural Muscles,"* American Journal of Physiology, Vol. 186, 1956

*"Industrial Injuries of the Back and Extremities,"* Journal of Bone and Joint Surgery, Vol. 54-A, No. 8, Dec. 1972

*"Intensive Exercises for the Low Back,"* by Iadore Brown, Physical Therapy, Vol. 50, No. 4, April 1970

*"Prevention of Low Back Pain,"* by Hans Kraus, M.D., Journal of Occupational Medicine, Nov. 1967

*"Cervical Spondylosis and Anterior Cervical Fusion,"* Surgery Annual, 1972

*"An Unorthodox Look at Backaches,"* by Joseph Tauber, Journal of Occupational Medicine, Vol. 12, April 1970

*"Application of the Overload Principle to Muscle Training in Man,"* American Journal of Physical Medicine, 1958